This book is due for return on or before the last date shown below.

Pain Management for
Health Professionals

Pain Management for Health Professionals

Pat O'Hara

Private occupational therapist

Consultant editor

Jo Campling

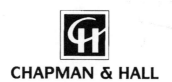

CHAPMAN & HALL

London • Weinheim • New York • Tokyo • Melbourne • Madras

Published by Chapman & Hall, 2–6 Boundary Row, London SE1 8HN, UK

Chapman & Hall, 2–6 Boundary Row, London SE1 8HN, UK

Chapman & Hall GmbH, Pappelallee 3, 69469 Weinheim, Germany

Chapman & Hall USA, 115 Fifth Avenue, New York NY 10003, USA

Chapman & Hall Japan, ITP-Japan, Kyowa Building, 3F, 2-2-1 Hirakawacho, Chiyoda-ku, Tokyo 102, Japan

Chapman & Hall Australia, 102 Dodds Street, South Melbourne, Victoria 3205, Australia

Chapman & Hall India, R. Seshadri, 32 Second Main Road, CIT East, Madras 600 035, India

Distributed in the USA and Canada by Singular Publishing Group Inc., 4284 41st Street, San Diego, California 92105

First edition 1996

© 1996 Pat O'Hara

Typeset in Great Britain by Saxon Graphics Ltd, Derby
Printed in Great Britain by St Edmundsbury Press, Bury St Edmunds, Suffolk

ISBN 0 412 62990 9   1 56593 436 9 (USA)

A catalogue record for this book is available from the British Library

∞ Printed on permanent acid-free text paper, manufactured in accordance with ANSI/NISO Z39.48-1992 and ANSI/NISO Z39.48-1984 (Permanence of Paper).

I would like to dedicate this book to Kevin, Adam, Liam and Kieran for their tolerance and support while it was being written.

Contents

Acknowledgements

I would like to thank the many students, both pre- and post-qualification, who have believed that I could write a book on pain management; the consultants I worked with at Gloucestershire Royal Hospital, who encouraged me to ask questions, write papers and increase my knowledge in this field; and the pain teams at Gloucestershire Royal Hospital, Gloucester and Input, St Thomas' Hospital, London. I would also like to thank my family for their support while this book was being written.

Introduction

This book is intended to provide a basic reference guide and information for those who are involved in the field of pain management. When teaching students, newly qualified staff and others who are just starting in pain management it has been difficult to identify one volume that would answer the beginner's needs.

I first became interested in pain management when confronted with a patient who developed thalamic pain four weeks post-stroke. The physiotherapist and myself were unable to carry out any treatment and there was little help or advice available to us at that time. We were told that thalamic pain was an unfortunate side effect of the stroke and was untreatable. We decided to treat the pain rather than the diagnosed condition, resulting in a reduction of pain which enabled us to carry out treatment. Following this episode I became interested in the treatment of pain and pain management and went on to work for five years in the pain management centre at Gloucestershire Royal Hospital in Gloucester.

Pain management is increasingly carried out in an interdisciplinary setting, resulting in shared information and a better understanding of the professional role of other disciplines. Guidelines are currently being drawn up for acute pain and pain management programmes. Education is also being addressed with the recent development of the Diploma in Pain Management at Cardiff and the introduction of pain management in both physiotherapy and occupational therapy training. I hope this book will enhance the reader's understanding in the rapidly developing field of pain management.

Physiology of pain 1

INTRODUCTION

Pain is a valuable and necessary part of the body's mechanism which usually indicates that something is wrong, for example tissue damage or disease. Pain can be caused by a variety of things, including injury, infection and inflammation. When pain is part of the disease process it provides information which can help in medical diagnosis, as it often has a characteristic pattern and presentation. Pain can also be secondary to treatment, diagnostic procedures or a process such as childbirth.

Pain enables the limb to be withdrawn from a painful stimulus, preventing further injury. Pain also acts as a basis for learning and prevents further injury or damage because the individual's pain experience indicates which objects or situations are potentially painful. Examples of this are being stung by a wasp and getting burnt by a hot object. When pain is caused by damage to the joints, infection or serious injury it can act as a limiting factor on activity. In this way the body ensures that the affected area of the body is rested so that healing can occur.

Components of pain

Even though the individual may have personal experience of pain and how it feels, they may still find it difficult to define and describe pain adequately. Although pain is unpleasant and usually associated with some type of injury, it also has several other components. It may be **sensory, affective** or **emotional, autonomic** or **motor** and each of these components may occur in isolation or in varying combinations and proportions (Halliday *et al.*, 1992).

The sensory component describes how the pain feels, i.e. it may be sharp, aching or related to the cause, e.g. burning, jabbing or stabbing. The affective or emotional component of pain refers to the emotional distress caused by the pain, i.e. 'it hurts'. The autonomic component relates to the changes which occur in the body, e.g. alteration in heart rate, blood pressure or body temperature when the body is under stress. The motor aspect refers to the withdrawal of the injured limb from the stimulus. This is known as a reflex and is often accompanied by vocalization and facial grimacing.

Pain usually arises from an obvious physical cause such as tissue damage or disease, however the relationship between the *stimulus* and its *response* is not always straightforward. For example, noxious stimuli do not always cause pain and the circumstances and psychological aspects also affect the response.

Transient, acute and chronic pain

Pain can be defined in three ways, as **transient**, **acute** and **chronic** (Melzack and Wall, 1991). Transient pain has a short duration and is the type of pain associated with a mild burn or stubbed toe. In this situation there is rarely any real damage to the limb and there is no associated anxiety. In transient pain there are two types of pain experienced. The first is mild and localized and is followed by a more diffuse intense pain, which may decrease in intensity or throb for several minutes before it fades away. These pains are commonly associated with minor injuries. However if the pain persists it may indicate that the toe is broken or the skin damaged by the heat and the pain is then said to be acute rather than transient.

Acute pain is characterized by a well defined time of onset and is associated with both subjective and objective signs indicating activation of the sympathetic nervous system (e.g. sweating, pallor, hypertension, grimacing). The individual experiences tissue damage, pain and related anxiety. The degree of anxiety experienced is dependent on the individual's experience and perception of the situation. Acute pain usually resolves once the cause is removed and healing has occurred, e.g. the type of pain associated with a sprained ankle. Again, the individual experiences two types of pain: initially sharp, well localized pain followed by a more diffuse widespread throbbing ache associated with swelling and inflammation of the damaged area.

Chronic pain persists long after healing has occurred, and is associated with both physiological and behavioural changes. At this stage the pain is not serving any useful function and may result in levels of activity and function being governed by the pain.

The function of pain is to alert the body to tissue injury before serious damage can occur and in this context it has both protective and survival value. Pain experience enables prevention of further damage by withdrawal or avoidance of the pain stimulus. Pain also promotes healing and recovery following injury as it limits activity, ensuring that the affected limb or area is rested. This promotes repair of the tissues and prevents further exacerbation of the injury.

LOCATION AND TYPES OF PAIN

Superficial or deep pain

Superficial pain occurs when the receptors in the surface tissues are stimulated, and it has a sharp, distinct quality. Deep pain comes from the deeper tissues and is duller, more persistent and less well located (Royle and Walsh, 1992). Deep pain is divided into **splanchnic pain**, occurring deep in the viscera, and **somatic pain**, which occurs in structures such as muscles, tendons, joints and periosteum. Pain in the visceral structures is poorly localized and builds up and reduces gradually. A feature of visceral pain is that it is referred to other parts of the body; for instance, cardiac pain is felt in the arm.

Localized or referred pain

Localized pain comes directly from the injury site, whereas referred pain is felt in a part of the body remote from the site of stimulation. Nerve impulses usually arise in an organ, with the pain being projected (or referred) to a surface area of the body. A classic example of referred pain is that associated with angina. The pain originates in the heart muscle as a result of ischaemia but may be experienced in the midsternal region, the base of the neck and down the left arm. This reflects the embryonic origins of the structures in the body. The heart originates in the neck of the embryo and receives its nerve supply from the cervical segments of the spinal cord. The embryonic link is maintained throughout development. Fibres carrying the pain messages from the viscera and the peripheral tissues converge upon the same neurone within the spinal cord.

Referred pain can also be secondary to reflex muscular spasm. The messages are interpreted as coming from superficial areas of the body because of previous pain experience (Royle and Walsh, 1992).

Projected pain

This occurs when pain messages are set up at a point along the pain pathway beyond the peripheral pain receptors (Royle and Walsh, 1992). An example of this is phantom limb pain following amputation. 'Stimuli coming from the stump may be localized on the basis of the previously established body image with the result that the pain is projected to the portion of the limb that was removed' (Royle and Walsh, 1992).

Intractable pain

This refers to any persistent, severe pain that cannot effectively be controlled by normal medication.

Psychogenic pain

This refers to pain for which there is no detectable organic lesion or peripheral stimulation. The discomfort is very real to the individual and is thought to be a physical manifestation of a psychological disturbance. Sternbach (1982) said that the term 'psychogenic pain' should only be applied to those patients who have no physical findings and a history of pain as an expression of their emotional problems. In the majority of chronic pain sufferers, pain can be related to a physical cause, with the behavioural and emotional factors influencing the individual's perception and expression of pain. Sternbach and Timmermans (1975) carried out studies with chronic pain patients undergoing treatment using the Minnesota Multiphasic Personality Inventory (MMPI). The results indicated that psychological factors are more likely to be caused by the chronic pain and will usually disappear or diminish following treatment of the pain.

PAIN RECEPTORS AND PAIN IMPULSE PATHWAYS

'Pain is the subjective manifestation of trauma transmitted by the sympathetic nervous system, which may interfere with normal functioning' (International Association for the Study of Pain, 1990).

Acute pain versus chronic pain

In the acute pain situation, e.g. a sprained ankle, a sharp pain is felt at the injury site. Tissue damage is detected by receptors, which have an axon-like process running from the periphery to the spinal cord. At the spinal cord it synapses with other cells carrying messages directly or indirectly to the brain.

Often the individual may try to alleviate the pain by rubbing or putting the limb under cold water. They are trying to **close the gate** to pain messages. Within 10 minutes of injury inflammation begins. The blood supply increases and serum begins to build up in the injured area. The protein contained in the serum eventually forms the healing fibrous tissue. In the short term this causes swelling in the area due to the large amount of serum produced. This results in a dull, aching throb, as the chemicals also stimulate other, slower nerve pain pathways. This swelling, combined with the pain experienced in this type of injury, makes it difficult to move and so rest is enforced, enabling healing to occur.

In long-term pain the receptors in the damaged tissue are repeatedly being stimulated. This may make the nociceptor very sensitive so that a light touch to the area may be mistakenly 'sent off' as a pain message. In this instance the pain message is not serving any useful purpose.

Pain receptors

In the skin, the muscles and around the joints there are specialized nerve endings that respond to various stimuli such as pain or heat. Sensory nerve endings that respond specifically to tissue damage are called **nociceptors**. Pain is a stimulus, not a feeling, and the receptors for pain are stimulated by various types of stimuli. As these receptors respond to noxious stimulation, which does not always elicit pain, the preferred terminology is nociceptor, not pain receptor (Halliday *et al.*, 1992). Many stimuli are non-specific but elicit pain through their intensity. For instance, light pressure produces an awareness of touch, but increasing the intensity of the pressure causes pain. Similarly, heat and cold must reach a certain intensity to stimulate nociceptors. Nociceptors are activated by intense stimulation and are sensitized by the presence of inflammation.

The nociceptive pathway starts with the stimulation of receptors, which are free nerve endings forming a diffuse network in the tissues. These receptors vary in concentration throughout the body. They are concentrated mainly in the skin and joint surfaces with only a few in the deeper tissues and viscera. Some nociceptors respond to specific stimuli, but many are polymodal, as they respond to any stimulus threatening tissue integrity. These nociceptors recognize force/pressure, temperature (that is varying pressure and temperature) and chemicals. When damage occurs, chemicals such as prostaglandins and kinins are released at the site of injury.

Nociceptor pathways

Nerve structure

The major nerves are large structures surrounded by their own sheath of connective tissue and special blood vessels. They are divided into bundles, surrounded by sheets of connective tissue. Each bundle contains large numbers of nerve fibres. Each nerve fibre is composed of a cell body, an **axon**, and dendrites. The axon is the basic structure that carries the nerve impulse and it also transports chemicals along its length. Each major nerve is a mixed nerve containing **motor**, **sensory** and **sympathetic** axons. The motor axons carry impulses which cause the muscles to contract. The sensory axons carry impulses which deliver afferent signals to the spinal cord, and the sympathetic axons carry impulses which control autonomic activities such as blood flow and sweating.

Sensory, or **afferent**, nerve fibres carry impulses to the **central nervous system** (**CNS**). Motor, or **efferent**, nerve fibres transmit impulses away from the central nervous system via the ventral nerve roots to the effector organs such as muscles. The afferent nerve fibres are divided into three groups, **A-delta**, **A-beta** and **C fibres**, and are classified according to the diameter and conduction velocity of the axon. The A fibres are surrounded by a fatty sheath (myelin). A-delta fibres have a conduction velocity of 5–36 m/s and are found in the mechanonociceptors, thermoreceptors for cold and mechanoreceptors. A-beta fibres have a conduction velocity of 36–90 m/s. They are found in the low-threshold mechanoreceptors and proprioceptors in joints and muscles. C fibres are unmyelinated, have a conduction velocity of 1–3 m/s and are found in the polymodal nociceptors, thermoreceptors and mechanoreceptors. A-beta fibres are activated by vibration and light touch, A-delta fibres by pinprick and C fibres by tissue damage (Carroll and Bowsher, 1995). The nociceptive afferents synapse with two main groups of neurons in the dorsal horn, specific nociceptor neurons and multimodal (non-specific) neurons. The latter receive many convergent inputs, including visceral afferents.

The initial sharp pain felt when trauma occurs is carried by the A-delta fibres, which transmit the impulses very quickly. This pain sensation is sharp, precise and easily localized. The C fibres conduct more slowly and have many connections, resulting in a throbbing, burning type of pain which is more diffuse and follows the initial sharp pain transmitted by the A-delta fibres. The A-beta fibres are activated when cutaneous stimulation, e.g. rubbing of the skin, occurs.

Pain impulses

Pain impulses are transmitted from the stimulus site by specific sensory nerve fibres which enter the spinal cord via the **dorsal** and **ventral** spinal roots. The impulses are then transmitted to neurones within the posterior column or horn of grey matter. Some impulses pass directly to motor neurons which initiate a reflex response, such as withdrawal of the injured part from the stimulus (e.g. the withdrawal of the hand from a very hot object). Other pain impulses cross to the opposite side of the cord and ascend via the **anterolateral spinothalamic** pathway to the brain. There are several pathways from the spinal cord to the brain. The spinothalamic tracts project to the somatosensory cortex and are thought to serve the sensory and discriminative aspects of pain. There is also a less specific pathway which is thought to involve the **spinoreticular** tract. The spinoreticular tract makes widespread and diffuse connections with many areas of the forebrain, including the limbic system, and is involved in the affective aspects of pain. The spinothalamic tract conveys specific information in relation to the qualities and location of the stimuli, whereas the spinoreticular tract conveys less specific information (Royle and Walsh, 1992; Halliday *et al.*, 1992).

Reflex response

A reflex is an automatic response: examples of this are the blink reflex when having a flash photograph taken or withdrawal of the hand or foot from a painful stimulus. The message is carried along the sensory pathway to the spinal cord, where it synapses with the efferent pathway, causing a response in a muscle or related structure. This circuit is called a **reflex arc**. When the receptors are stimulated impulses are transmitted along the sensory nerves to the CNS where they synapse with the intermediate (internuncial) neurones, which then synapse with the efferent or motor neurones that relay messages back to the periphery to the effectors. The effectors are the glands or muscles that carry out the response, e.g. the knee jerk reflex. The cell bodies of sensory neurones are located in the dorsal root ganglion and the internuncial cell bodies are contained in the grey matter. The efferent fibres exit via the ventral roots of the dorsal horn.

Pain control

In 1965 Melzack and Wall put forward the gate control theory in an effort to explain the mechanisms which can inhibit the transmission of pain messages. The basic concept is that, when the afferent neurons are stimulated, the pathway can be blocked or filtered by a synaptic 'gate' in the dorsal horn of the spinal cord. This gate is thought to be located in the substantia gelatinosa of the dorsal horn. The neurons of the substantia gelatinosa have connections with the primary afferent fibres and the dorsal horn cells (Chapter 2). In addition to this gating mechanism the **endogenous analgesic systems** are also activated by nociceptor inputs. There are three known components:

- Descending pathways
- Opioid receptors
- Endogenous analgesics.

Descending pathways

In the 1970s experiments were carried out using electrical stimulation of the **periaqueductal grey matter** (PAGM), this produced analgesia and was known as **stimulation-produced analgesia (SPA)**. Mayer *et al.* (1971) researched this extensively in experiments with rats and found that the effects were confined to specific areas of skin and that SPA lasted for a few minutes following the cessation of the stimulus. Electrical stimulation also appears to activate some of the neural systems that modulate nociceptive information. The descending pathways from the PAGM are able to exert inhibitory control over nociceptive responses at the level of the dorsal horn and possibly trigger the gate control mechanism.

Opioid receptors

When a harmful stimulus activates the nociceptors and ascending fibres the analgesic system is activated. This involves special receptors called opiate receptors situated in the midbrain PAGM, the costroventral medulla and the dorsal horns of the spinal cord. In 1973 Pert and Snyder demonstrated the presence of opioid receptors in the brain tissue. Three types of opioid receptor site have been identified and these have practical application for the effective use of opioid analgesics such as morphine. Opioid analgesics chemically bind to these receptors in order to work.

Endogenous analgesics

Snyder (1977) identified a substance called **endorphin**. Endorphins are released by impulses from the brain and bind with narcotic receptors located at nerve endings in the brain and spinal cord. Endogenous analgesics such as enkephalins and endorphins are produced by the brain and have a similar action to morphine. **Enkephalins** are found in the areas of the brain and spinal cord associated with pain control, the dorsal horn and the substantia gelatinosa. They are short-acting and act at the synaptic level. Endorphins are found in the pituitary gland and the hypothalamus and are longer-acting. Enkephalins and endorphins appear to function as excitatory transmitter substances which have an inhibitory effect on the nociceptive pathway that closes the pain gate. Endorphin levels vary between individuals and levels can be depleted by factors such as prolonged pain, stress, alcohol and drugs. Levels can be raised by exercise, trauma, acupuncture and some types of nerve stimulation.

The endogenous analgesic system can be activated as part of the stress response and many forms of physical stress, such as exercise, eating, drinking and sexual behaviour, are known to cause the release of enkephalins and endorphins When the 'fight or flight' aspects of the stress response are activated, which involve the release of adrenal hormones and increased sympathetic response, the pain can effectively be 'turned off'. The explorer David Livingstone (Melzack and Wall, 1991) reported that when he was attacked by a lion and shaken like 'a terrier with a rat', he felt no pain and was conscious of what was happening. This is an example of the increased stress response causing activation of the endogenous analgesic system and effectively turning off the pain.

ACUTE PAIN

Acute pain subsides as healing takes place and it has a predictable end (McCaffery and Beebe, 1989). The duration of acute pain is brief and is usually defined as less than 3 months. Pain is a very complex phenomenon, as several components – affective, autonomic, motor and sensory – are involved in the pain response. It is also subjective and has quantifiable features such as intensity, quality, duration and personal meaning to the individual. The individual's perception of the pain is influenced by their previous experience and cultural upbringing. Acute pain usually refers to pain that is sudden in onset and severe but it can also be slow in onset, e.g. headaches. Pain intensity can vary from mild to severe.

Physiological aspects

The physiological responses that occur when the nociceptors are stimulated are similar to those of the stress response or 'fight or flight' response. The sympathetic system is activated, increasing the heart rate and respiratory rate and raising the blood pressure. Other symptoms that people complain of are sweating, churning of the stomach, coldness and nausea. The sympathetic system causes general vasoconstriction but dilates the arteries supplying vital organs such as the muscles. The sympathetic system is activated in an emergency situation and diverts the blood supply to areas of the body where it will be needed for a fight or flight situation.

Psychological aspects

The reaction to pain differs between individuals and research has been carried out to ascertain whether this is caused by inherited differences or environmental factors.

The influence of development and learning

In the 1950s Melzack carried out experiments with puppies who were raised in isolation (Melzack and Wall, 1965). At maturity these dogs displayed abnormal behaviour towards noxious stimuli such as a lighted match. They did not have any affective reaction such as cowering or whimpering, although they exhibited the normal reflex withdrawal from the match. Other pups from the litter, raised under normal conditions, quickly learned the potential danger of the lighted match. When young animals are reared under normal circumstances they learn about different environmental stimuli through play, exploration and fighting. Melzack also found a difference between breeds who were raised in isolation. Beagles raised in isolation exhibited more normal behaviour than Scotties or mongrels, suggesting that heredity may influence the extent to which early experience modifies behaviour. Although there is some evidence to suggest that heredity does influence the way we react to a stimuli there is also evidence to suggest that early experience affects the perception of pain.

Pavlov (1927, 1928) found that even established reactions to a particular stimulus could be altered. He carried out experiments with dogs that involved conditioning to a stimulus, i.e. the presentation of food following the application of an electrical shock to the paw. Eventually the dogs would salivate as a reaction to the electric shock without the food being presented. This illustrates how reflexes can be altered and modified by conditioning. It also demonstrates that any peripheral stimulation is identified, localized and evaluated prior to the input of perception and experience which influences the ensuing behaviour. Pain thresholds and tolerances can be affected by culture and experience; however there is little evidence to suggest that any difference is due to genetic influences.

American women of Italian descent are reported to have a lower tolerance to electric shock than women of northern European or Jewish origin. This difference is more likely to be due to factors following birth than genetic factors. For instance, women of Italian origin are more expressive than their northern European counterparts. Interaction with the family group influences these responses. The mother's initial response to a situation can reinforce or modify subsequent behaviour of the child.

Is there a pain personality?

Psychiatric illnesses or emotional disturbances can exhibit pain as a symptom but this does not prove that there is a relationship between pain and personality. Many studies have been carried out on this topic and the relationship between pain and personality appears to be a complex one. Although personality can affect our perception of pain, equally pain experience can influence personality. Bond and Pearson (1969) investigated the incidence of pain and the relationship with personality in women with cervical cancer. The women were divided into three groups. Group I had no pain, Group 2 had pain but were not receiving medication and Group 3 had pain and were receiving medication. The Eysenck Personality Inventory was used to assess each woman's personality. There was no significant difference in the mean scores of the experimental group (i.e. Groups 1, 2 and 3) and the control group. However, there were differences between Groups 1, 2 and 3. The pain-free group (Group 1) and those who were on medication (Group 3) were scored as extroverts and the group who were in pain but did not receive medication (Group 2) were scored as introverts. Levels of neuroticism were higher in Groups 2 and 3, with Group 2 being the highest. However this cannot be related to pre-existing personality traits as there was no information relating to the women's personality prior to the onset of their illness. Bond stated that following successful surgery mean neuroticism scores were reduced.

Any personality change associated with illness or pain is also dependent on the nature of the clinical condition. Generally, acute pain is associated with anxiety but chronic pain is more likely to be associated with depression.

Disorders associated with both acute and chronic pain

The following are some common disorders associated with pain. However, this list is neither exclusive nor exhaustive.

Ankylosing spondylitis

Ankylosing spondylitis predominantly occurs in young adults. This disease causes the joints and ligaments of the spine to harden gradually and become calcified. Eventually the spine becomes stiff and inflexible, resulting in a flat chest and flexed spine. The inflammation process that occurs during the progress of the disease causes pain and discomfort, as does the resulting stiffness of the joints and ligaments. In many cases this condition is considered to be a chronic pain condition.

Arachnoiditis

This is usually caused by the inflammation of the inner lining or dural sheath within the spinal canal. Arachnoiditis was a rare complication of investigative procedures such as myelograms, when an oil-based contrast was used. Modern techniques use a water-based contrast and this complication no longer occurs. A mild infection or inflammation caused by bleeding near the exposed dural sheath may sometimes cause arachnoiditis after discectomy operation. In many cases this becomes a chronic pain condition.

Cancer pain

A tumour or cancer can invade an organ or the spine and develop in it, causing pressure on surrounding tissues and nerves. Studies suggest that moderate to severe pain is experienced by one-third of cancer patients receiving active therapy, and by 60–80% of patients with advanced cancer (Bonica, 1980). Pain can be caused by bone metastases and by compression or infiltration of nervous structures, veins, arteries and lymphatics. Obstruction of areas such as the bowel can cause pain, as can ulceration of pain-sensitive mucosal surfaces. Treatment processes such as surgery, chemotherapy and radiation therapy can also cause pain. Some pain is caused by the general debility of the patient, joint stiffness, pressure sores and constipation. Cancer pain can become chronic in the later stages of the condition.

Gall bladder problems

Gall stones and inflammation of the gall bladder are usually accompanied by colicky pain in the abdomen and sometimes nausea and vomiting. Pain is sometimes referred to below the shoulder blade and may be accompanied by fever and shaking.

Gynaecological problems

Referred pain to the lower back is often associated with disorders of the female reproductive organs such as womb prolapse. Back pain is also associated with menstruation, uterine cramps and premenstrual tension. Backache, abdominal pain, vaginal discharge and pain during intercourse are associated with infections of the uterus or fallopian tubes.

Heart attack

The pain is severe, is located in the chest and may spread up to the jaw or down one arm. The pain may also be felt in the back, though it is never confined to the back. The pain is accompanied by symptoms of nausea, dizziness, shortness of breath and palpitations.

Inflammation of the pancreas

This manifests itself as an intermittent gnawing pain in the back and attacks are usually related to alcoholic intake.

Influenza and other fevers

Influenza normally starts with a feeling of general malaise, mild fever and wide-spread aches and pains. The main symptoms are usually fever and headache, often accompanied by a stiff painful neck if there is a high fever.

Kidney problems

Kidney stones can cause intermittent colicky pain in the lower back, and nausea. The pain is caused by a blockage in the tube from the kidney to the bladder, causing pain in the groin area. This is often accompanied by a kidney infection.

Pneumonia and pleurisy

Pain occurs around the lower ribs and towards the back and may be the first symptom of a lung infection. Pain may be referred to the shoulders and is often associated with breathing in.

Rheumatoid arthritis

Inflammation in various joints of the body, as in rheumatoid arthritis, can cause pain and discomfort. It usually starts in the small joints of the hands and feet and progresses until it affects the larger joints, such as knees, hips, elbows and shoulders. Osteoarthritis predominantly affects the hips, knees and interphalangeal joints and is a degenerative joint disorder, whereas rheumatoid arthritis is a chronic systemic disease. Many people are told that they have arthritis by their doctor, especially when discussing back conditions. However the doctor is usually referring to the normal signs of wear and tear associated with ageing, not rheumatoid arthritis. This condition can be classed as acute or chronic in relation to pain.

Stomach ulcer

Ulcers may cause a severe burning pain in the back; this is usually worse following a fatty or spicy meal.

Others

Acute pain can also occur postoperatively, and with bony fractures and strepto-coccal throat infections.

CHRONIC PAIN

'Because the link between pain and injury is easy to see it is believed that pain is always the result of physical damage and that the intensity of the pain we feel is proportional to the severity of injury' (Melzack and Wall, 1991).

Defining chronic pain

Chronic pain is defined as pain that persists for longer than 3 months which recurs on a regular basis or is ongoing on a daily basis. The onset is less well defined than acute pain and the cause is usually non-life-threatening (McCaffery and Beebe, 1989). Chronic pain is a complex physiological and psychological phenomenon that causes varying degrees of disability. It can start as acute pain but persist over an extended period of time. The pain may be mild, moderate or severe and can be intermittent or continuous. The cause may be unknown and even if it is known is unlikely to be altered by conventional approaches using the medical model. The associated alterations in an individual's lifestyle and function often lead to anxiety states, depression and general debility. McCaffery and Beebe classify chronic pain as recurrent, chronic acute or chronic non-malignant pain.

Recurrent pain

Migraine headaches are an example of recurrent pain. They are episodic with a predicted end, but have a tendency to recur. In between episodes the sufferer is usually pain-free although the rate of recurrence may be frequent, i.e. weekly or monthly.

Chronic acute pain

Chronic acute pain can last for months or years and, although it does not have a predictable time span, it is likely to end. Occurrence is usually daily over a long period. Examples of this type of pain are cancer and burn pain.

Chronic non-malignant pain

This is also called chronic benign pain. The individual is disabled by the pain and may be diagnosed as having chronic intractable benign pain syndrome. The recurrence rate is daily and lasts for longer than 3 months. The intensity may vary, from mild to very severe. Causation is usually attributed to non-life-threatening causes and the pain does not respond to treatment. The pain has no predictable end. Examples of this condition are phantom limb pain, peripheral neuropathy and Raynaud's disease. With long-term pain problems the body's responses can change. For example if the nerve receptors are repeatedly stimulated they can become sensitized so that they respond to a signal of light touch as though they have been injured. The message is being relayed to the brain although there is no new damage to the tissues or joint. In other words, although the cause of the original pain has been treated or removed, the pain message is still being transmitted along the pathway.

Lifestyle

Chronic pain can influence the activity levels of the individual. Many pain sufferers are not able to perform everyday tasks such as housework or cooking and they may need help with self-care activities such as dressing and bathing. The commonest changes to lifestyle are having to give up work due to pain, a reduced level of housework or social activity and a loss of role and self-esteem.

The pain sufferer often has a lifestyle of overactivity (doing too much) and underactivity caused by this. This leads to a routine of frequent rests during the day and avoidance of situations, people and any activities which cause stress or pain. There is a general withdrawal from social activity and life becomes governed by the pain. Chronic pain causes endorphin depletion, which in turn results in decreased pain perception and tolerance thresholds. When pain is persistent it can cause poor sleep patterns and a loss of appetite, often resulting in a general fatigue, malaise and disability. If the pain is not controlled it may cause a disruption of family, work and social life. Pain sufferers are often on high doses of medication, are drinking or smoking more and have sleep problems. The physiological changes associated with chronic pain can lead to inefficient functioning and increased psychological responses to pain (O'Hara, 1990).

Psychological response

The psychological response to pain is influenced by the individual's previous experience and the degree of threat and frustration related to the pain. Some people express their emotions and feelings associated with the pain vocally or through non-verbal behaviour, while others may 'suffer in silence'. Because of social isolation, loss of role and the inability to do things, people often get depressed. They can see no point in making plans and have nothing to look forward to. Depression often accompanies inactivity and creates a new set of problems. Often the person feels frustrated and a failure. This leads to a lack of motivation and desire to do things. Sleep may be disturbed, often leading to a reliance on sleeping tablets (O'Hara, 1990). Research has also shown that depression increases the perception of pain.

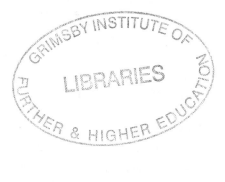

<table>
<tr><td>

2

</td><td>

Pain theory

</td></tr>
</table>

HISTORY OF PAIN THEORY

Specificity theory

The traditional theory of pain is known as '**specificity theory**'. This theory proposed that a specific pain system carried messages from the pain receptors in the skin to a pain centre in the brain. A description of this theory was provided by Descartes (1664). He saw the pain system as a direct link between the periphery of the body and special areas in the brain. According to Descartes this could be likened to the bell-ringing mechanism in a church. When the bell rope is pulled the bell rings in the tower. The relationship between pain and injury was thought to be directly proportional. In other words, pain associated with a minor cut gives minimal discomfort whereas pain associated with major trauma hurts a lot.

Muller (1842) stated that the brain received information about external objects by way of the sensory nerves, and proposed the **doctrine of specific nerve energies**. He only recognized the five classical senses – seeing, hearing, taste, smell and touch. His concept was that of a direct pathway from the sensory organ to the relevant area in the cortical centres of the brain, namely the auditory or visual cortex. In the late 19th and early 20th centuries nerve impulses were perceived to be the same in all sensory nerves. This resulted in a search for a terminal centre in the brain for each sensory nerve.

In 1920 Head proposed that the thalamus contained the pain centre and that the cortex was able to exert inhibitory control over it. Von Frey (Boring, 1942) elaborated on Muller's theory and stated that there were four sensory modalities: touch, cold, warmth and pain. He also identified a separate centre for each modality, located in the brain. Specificity theorists stated that there were two types of fibres for pain, the A-delta fibre and the C fibre, and in 1957 Keele established that the pain pathway followed the ascending spinothalamic tract. However, psychological evidence does not support the proposed relationship between pain perception and intensity of the stimulus stated in the specificity theories. Clinically, conditions such as phantom limb pain, neuralgias and causalgia do not conform to the concept of a direct-route nervous system.

Pattern theories

Peripheral pattern theory

In 1955 Weddell considered that pain was due to excessive peripheral stimulation of non-specific receptors and that the resulting patterns of nerve impulses were interpreted centrally as pain. This was based on the assumption that all nerve endings (apart from those that innervate hair cells) are similar. This is refuted by the physiological evidence, which has shown that there is a high degree of receptor-fibre specialization.

Central summation theory

Livingston (1943) suggested that there were specific central neural mechanisms which could be used as an explanation for pain phenomena such as phantom limb pain, causalgia and neuralgias. 'He proposed that the initial damage to the limb, or the trauma associated with its removal, initiates abnormal firing patterns in reverberatory circuits in the dorsal horns of the spinal cord, which send volleys of nerve impulses to the brain, giving rise to pain' (Melzack and Wall, 1991). This may spread to adjoining neurons in the lateral and ventral horns, producing autonomic and muscular reactions such as sweating and jerky movements in the stump. This mechanism increases the sensory input causing a 'vicious circle' between the central and peripheral processes, which perpetuate this abnormal spinal activity. When this occurs, even light touch will trigger these abnormal reactions.

Sensory interaction theory

This theory proposes that there are two fibre systems, a myelinated and an unmyelinated system (Noordenbos, 1959). Synaptic transmission is inhibited in the unmyelinated system (which carries the signals for pain) by the myelinated system. It also proposes that damage to the myelinated system leads to pathological pain states. In pathological conditions the myelinated system becomes less dominant, causing a diffuse burning pain or hyperalgesia. Noordenbos stated that if the fibres carrying the impulses which produce pain are greater than those inhibiting the pain there is increased neural transmission and therefore increased pain levels. The spinal cord was seen as a multisynaptic afferent system with diffuse connections giving many alternative avenues for impulses to be transmitted to the brain.

Affect theory of pain

Pain as a sensory modality is a recent concept: people like Aristotle saw pain as the opposite of pleasure. Even in 1939, Dallenbach considered pain to be an emotion rather than a sensation. Marshall (1894), who was a philosopher and psychologist, stated that 'pain is an emotional quality that colours all sensory events'. He felt that pain had to be more than a sensation as it also had qualities of negative affect which could spur us into action. Pain causes us to carry out actions in order to stop the pain and this type of behaviour is both motivational and emotional.

During the 20th century pain has become accepted as a sensory modality. However, the affect theory of pain is still incomplete as an explanation of pain mechanisms. It does not take into account the fact that sensory, motivational and cognitive processes occur in parallel and are interacting systems.

PAIN THEORY TODAY

The theories discussed in the previous sections do not explain why the pain experienced can have little or no relationship to the severity of the injury. Neither do they explain why pain can occur in the absence of damage to the body or why surgical interruption of the central pathways can fail to relieve pain either partially or on a permanent basis. The following sections look more closely at these aspects.

Does injury occur without pain?

Pain is often believed to be the result of physical damage and the intensity of pain experienced is expected to be proportional to the severity of the injury. In general this is true: a minor injury such as knocking the arm on a cupboard results in mild pain experienced for a few seconds. But, if the individual is knocked down in a road accident, the pain is excruciating and lasts for longer. However this is not always the case. Some people are born without the ability to feel pain even when they are injured seriously (**congenital analgesia**) and many people have injuries, for example cuts and bruises, where pain is not felt until minutes or hours have passed. This is known as **episodic analgesia**. There are also pains that have no association with known tissue damage or that persist even though the injury site appears to have healed. This illustrates how variable the link between pain and injury is – 'Injury may occur without pain, and pain without injury' (Melzack and Wall, 1991).

Congenital analgesia

Many people who have congenital analgesia suffer from burns, bruises and lacerations in childhood. They have been known to bite their tongues while chewing food and have to learn how to avoid inflicting severe wounds on themselves. Other problems arise when they break a limb and they have been known to walk on a leg with a hairline fracture until the limb fractures completely. They are also at risk from kidney infections, ruptured appendix, etc. as they are unable to feel the severe pain that normally accompanies these disorders. When examined there does not appear to be any abnormality of the nervous system. 'It is as though the system is not switched on' (Melzack and Wall, 1991).

One of the documented examples is that of a Canadian, Miss C., who was a student at a university in Montreal in the 1950s. Her father was a doctor and was aware of her problems and asked colleagues in Montreal to examine her. Miss C. was intelligent and normal in every way except that she seemed unable to feel pain. In childhood she had bitten off the tip of her tongue while eating and suffered third-degree burns when she knelt on a hot radiator to look out of a window. She was unable to feel pain when experiencing electric shock, hot water or a prolonged icebath. Her gag reflex was elicited with difficulty and she did not appear to be able to sneeze or cough. Miss C. had many pathological changes in her joints as she did not have any protection – i.e. pain sensation. Because she was unable to experience discomfort or pain she did not transfer her weight when standing or turn over in bed to avoid pressure or certain positions. Miss C. died at the age of 29 from osteomyelitis (Melzack and Wall, 1991).

When nerves that normally innervate a joint are missing or defective the joint surfaces become damaged and the ligaments and other tissues are stretched. The blood supply is reduced and the area becomes prone to infection. Persistent injury and damage to joints is apparent, especially, in those joints that are normally subject to minor injury, i.e. ankles, knees, wrists and elbows. These are known as Charcot joints. This condition is also seen following diabetic neuropathy.

Comings and Amromin (1974), found that congenital analgesia can be due to many causes. Sometimes there is evidence of neurological damage; this occurs in a disorder called dysautonomia or Riley–Day syndrome. All physical development is abnormal and the people rarely live to adulthood. Other documented causes are the inability to sweat and mental retardation. When people are insensitive to pain they do not recognize symptoms of appendicitis, breaking of limbs, burns, cuts and bruises. As a consequence people with this condition have to learn to avoid injury and to recognize other signs of illness such as loss of appetite. Congenital analgesia is a rare condition but it illustrates the important role that pain plays in survival.

Episodic analgesia

Episodic analgesia, is seen more often. This is when one experiences pain many minutes or hours after the injury, which can range from minor cuts and bruises to broken bones or loss of a limb. Beecher (1959) documented the behaviour of soldiers severely wounded in battle in the Second World War. Only one in three complained of enough pain to require morphine. Many denied having pain or said they had so little that they did not require medication. However they could feel pain, as they felt the vein being punctured when blood was taken. Beecher considered that the failure to feel pain from their wounds was due to the feeling of relief or euphoria at having escaped death on the battlefield despite their injury.

Carlen *et al.* (1978) carried out a study with Israeli soldiers who had traumatic amputations after the Yom Kippur War. They found similar results. In a more recent study (Melzack, Wall and Ty, 1982) it was found that 37% of people arriving at an Accident and Emergency clinic with a variety of injuries (which included amputated fingers, major lacerations and fractures) reported that they did not feel pain until minutes or even hours after the injury. There are also instances of people being able to lie on beds of nails, walk on burning coals and put needles into their flesh without apparently causing pain.

The characteristics of episodic analgesia are that the condition has no relation to the severity or location of the injury and the injured person is fully aware of the nature of the injury and its consequences. The meaning the individual ascribes to the situation can affect their perception of the pain and consequently its effect. There also appears to be an element of attention distraction involved, but not in every case. Analgesia is instantaneous, has a limited time-span and is localized to the injury site.

Does pain occur without injury?

There are several conditions in which pain is experienced by people without any apparent injury. These include common complaints such as tension headaches and migraine.

Headaches

People can develop pain without apparent injury, as in, for example, tension headaches. These are widely believed to be caused by muscle tension but work carried out by Pikoff (1984) found that the muscles were not found to be contracted. Similarly, migraines have been thought to be caused by dilated blood vessels in the head but research by Olesen (1986) has shown that changes in the blood vessels are the results of headaches rather than the cause. There is no real evidence to support the theory that migraines and headaches are caused by anxiety and tension, but they can enhance the pain.

Trigeminal neuralgia

In trigeminal neuralgia stabbing pain can be caused by light touch to a trigger point. Studies of the tissues and nerves have shown them to be normal. Excruciating pain can be triggered in both migraine and trigeminal neuralgia by the application of innocuous stimuli such as warmth or gentle touch. It is likely that abnormal information processing in the CNS is the cause of this phenomenon. There are many inputs that cause these conditions and they do not occur in isolation. The cutaneous input may be accompanied by sympathetic activity as well as input from the visual and auditory systems. The pain may occur spontaneously and may have a long duration.

Low back pain

Similarly, in patients with low back pain diagnostic techniques may reveal no evidence of damage. Work carried out by Loeser (1980) found no damage in 70% of cases. Relief of back pain by surgery may have a success rate as low as 60%. In studies carried out by Loeser (1980) and Watts (1985) the researchers found that over half of the patients who suffer back pain were symptom-free within a month without any intervention. Therapies such as behaviour modification, relaxation, hypnosis and biofeedback have been used in the treatment of back pain and have been shown to help some patients. Swanson *et al.* (1976) carried out work with a group of patients, predominantly with low back pain, using a variety of techniques. A total of 80% were found to have marked to moderate improvement following treatment, and 50% continued to improve 3–6 months later. More recent research based on controlled outcome studies (Bonica, 1990) indicates that multidisciplinary pain management programmes are more effective than individual treatment by a single discipline (Chapter 10).

Kidney stone

Sometimes, pain can appear to be out of all proportion to the severity of the causative event, e.g. the passing of a kidney stone. This results in extreme pain, caused by peristaltic contractions. The patient presents as pale, with a rapid pulse, knees drawn into the body, and a rigid abdominal wall due to the pain. However, the passing of a kidney stone is a minor event in an area that is poorly innervated in comparison with the skin. There is no apparent explanation for the pain being so severe. When the stone is passed into the bladder, relief is complete and instantaneous.

Pain may persist long after healing has occurred

Phantom limb pain

Wynn Parry (1980) carried out a study consisting of 100 cases of brachial plexus avulsion injury in motorcycle accidents. In these cases the arm was paralysed from the shoulder down, there was muscle wasting and total anaesthesia of the arm. In the study, 95 patients reported that they could feel a normal arm but that it felt as though it did not belong to them. The phantom limb was also extremely painful, the whole arm feeling as though it was on fire.

Damage of peripheral nerves in the arms or legs, by gunshot wounds or other injuries, can also give rise to excruciating pain that persists long after the tissues have healed. They are often described as burning, cramping or shooting pains. Not only can injury occur without pain but excruciating pain can be experienced in the absence of apparent injury and it can also arise in parts of the body that have been removed. Some amputees may suffer periodic pain episodes, either daily or weekly, whereas others may have pain continuously. Pain onset can be immediately post-amputation or may not occur for weeks, months or even years after the amputation. It is as if the limb is being held in an uncomfortable position with the muscles in constant contraction.

Causalgia

The characteristics of causalgia are an intense burning pain in the area innervated by a damaged nerve. Although there is a loss of sensitivity in this area once the pain is triggered the burning pain continues after the stimulus is withdrawn and is often intense in nature. Mitchell (1872) described this condition in relation to bullet injuries in the American Civil War. Livingston (1943) also described it in relation to military casualties. Evidence now suggests that causalgic pain can follow any peripheral nerve injury including damage by fracture, cancer and multiple sclerosis. (Noordenbos, 1959; Schott 1986). Causalgic pain can occur immediately the injury is sustained or weeks or months later. The area of abnormal sensitization can spread to include skin not innervated by the damaged nerve. Eventually even small movements or vibrations can trigger the pain.

Surgical interruption of pathways

Doctors originally thought that if they cut the nerves carrying the pain messages, this would get rid of the pain. Unfortunately they found that this did not work, as the pain messages found other routes. For example, when someone has a below-knee amputation the nerves to the toes are severed. The person may still be able to feel phantom limb pain in the toes that have been amputated. There are many areas higher up in the system that send messages to try and 'close the gate' to pain, but these are unable to function in this situation, as the descending pathway is also severed. Jensen *et al.* (1983, 1985) carried out studies with amputees. They found that 72% had phantom limb pain 8 days after amputation and 65% still had phantom limb pain 6 months later. Various operations have been carried out for interruption of peripheral nerves, dorsal roots and the spinothalamic tracts (Chapter 6). These may provide some relief initially but the pain usually returns often worse than before.

Social and psychological influences on pain

Beecher (1956) compared the level of medication required following severe trauma in soldiers and civilians. The civilian group requested medication more often than the soldiers. He concluded that the difference between the groups was mediated by psychological factors. The soldiers' relief at escaping from the front line was greater than the pain from the injury – i.e. they saw their injury in a positive light – whereas the civilian saw their wounds as preventing them from working, putting them at a financial disadvantage, i.e. in a negative light.

Other research has found that if the individual is able to exercise control in the pain situation their response can be affected. Mowrer and Vick (1948) carried out experiments with laboratory rats who were given electric shocks while eating. The group who had some control over the situation ate more and were less disturbed. Hokanson et al. (1971) carried out a similar study with human subjects. One group were able to take time out whenever they wished from the shock. The group with no control over their situation had a raised blood pressure. This reflected the differences in the subject's perception of the stimulus and the situation. Staub, Tursky and Schwartz (1971) carried out similar experiments: the subjects who had control over the situation had a reduced heart rate response to the electric shocks and rated the pain level lower than the other group. The group without control over the level of the shocks showed a lower tolerance than the group with control. In a further experiment the control was removed from the first group (the group who had control). They exhibited an increased perception of the pain and their tolerance levels were reduced.

Work has also been carried out on the use of placebos in pain reduction. Beecher (1959) found that, in post-surgical pain, relief was obtained when placebos were administered. Polgar and Thomas (1991) stated that the placebo effect was when an innocuous intervention resulted in either improvement of the condition or improvement in the patient's perception of their condition. This treatment benefited between 35% and 40% of patients. It has been found that placebo effects are applicable to surgery as well as medication and that the relief level experienced by the patient undergoing surgery was directly related to the surgeons conviction or enthusiasm. This would indicate that suggestion can promote pain reduction in certain situations for some patients.

Cultural influences

There is evidence to support the view that social and cultural factors influence the way we perceive or interpret pain. Melzack and Wall (1991) tell of the hook-swinging ritual practised in parts of India. One of the men is selected for the role of blessing the children and crops in the villages. He has steel hooks inserted under the skin and the muscle on his back and ropes are attached to the hooks. He is then suspended by the ropes from a beam on a cart and is driven from village to village. Despite the fact that the man is only suspended by the hooks he appears to feel no pain. Laboratory studies of pain tolerance also endorse the fact that there are differences between cultural and ethnic groups. Indian fakirs walk across beds of hot coals and lie on beds of nails with no obvious signs of pain. Studies on this phenomenon showed that the fakir needed two hours of concentration before entering his trance state (Larbig, 1982). When this was monitored on an encephalogram there were signs of increased mental activity and the sympathetic nervous system was geared for action not relaxation. When the fakir was lying on nails, walking on burning coals or piercing his body with swords and daggers there was no pain or bleeding.

Distraction

Studies have been carried out on attention and distraction. It has been found that if the individual's attention is directed towards a potentially painful event the severity of the pain will increase. Distraction, on the other hand, can reduce or alleviate the pain experience. Hall and Stride (1954) found that the appearance of the word 'pain' in instructions influenced the individual's reporting of the level of pain. When children fall and hurt themselves parents use distraction as part of the comforting process. In a survey by Niven (1986) it was found that distraction activities were most often used as coping strategies. Affleck *et al.* (1984) cited distraction as one of the principal occupational interventions for pain. The type of distraction used ranged from hobbies and games to guided imagery techniques. The use of these techniques resulted in a decreased perception of the pain and increased awareness and involvement of their environment. Research carried out in the laboratory situation would suggest that distraction is not always effective and only works when the pain is mild and short-lived. Other researchers have also found that distraction techniques work best if they involve increased attentional capacity and are used for mild rather than intense pain (McCaul and Mallott, 1984).

Summary of clinical evidence

In the above conditions the pain is unlikely to be attributable to a single cause. Inputs are received cutaneously, sympathetically and from the auditory and visual systems. These inputs act on the central nervous system, which produces impulse patterns that result in pain. Other factors that affect these conditions are anxiety, cognitions and emotions. The pain may be triggered by touch, heat or cold and may be mild or severe. It is thought that this pain phenomenon is due to abnormal information processing in the central nervous system. These pain conditions often persist long after the expected time for regeneration or healing to occur. Phantom limb pain may persist for many years and it is suggested that, as the pain frequently occurs at the site where injury or disease occurred prior to amputation, it is due to a pain memory mechanism. The area affected by the pain and trigger zones may increase over time to cover parts of the body unrelated to the original injury or pain site. This would indicate that there is a wide distribution of neural mechanisms which do not reflect dermatomal innervation of the body by the somatic nerves. The fact that the use of surgery to abolish pain frequently fails would also appear to endorse this.

PAIN GATE THEORY

In the 1960s Melzack and Wall proposed the **gate control theory**. This states that within the spinal cord there are factors that may block or close the gate to pain messages, but equally there are factors that open up the gate and make us more aware of the pain. The neural mechanisms in the dorsal horn of the spinal cord act like a gate, regulating the effects of afferent pathways on neurones in the CNS. Melzack and Wall felt that this new theory should explain why the relationship between injury and pain is so variable and why the location of pain can be different from the site of injury. It should also explain how pain can persist in the absence of injury or after healing and why the nature and location of pain can change over time. Finally the theory should explain why there is no adequate treatment for certain types of pain and why pain is multidimensional.

When injury occurs the A-delta fibres and the C fibres are stimulated. They deliver impulses, directly and indirectly, to the transmission cells in the spinal cord, which in their turn transmit to local reflex circuits and to the brain.

The synaptic junctions in the central nervous system (CNS) are complex and include cells that both facilitate and inhibit the flow of impulses. After an impulse is received by the cells in the dorsal horn of the spinal cord a prolonged burst of impulses is fired (Wall, 1960). All synaptic regions contain both inhibitory and excitatory mechanisms, which control transmission depending on the balance of activity. Cells located within the CNS can inhibit the afferent pain impulses, thereby closing the gate. This area is called the substantia gelatinosa and it contains both inhibitory and excitatory interneurons. The opening and closing of the gate is controlled by the activity patterns in other afferent inputs to the spinal cord and the descending pathways from the brain stem.

Both pre- and postsynaptic inhibition can occur. Cutaneous impulses stimulated by vibration, cold or heat are transmitted by A-beta fibres in the afferent nerve and these impulses can effectively block the impulses carried by the A-delta and C fibres, closing the pain gate. When a minor injury occurs, e.g. hitting the elbow or finger, the individual's reaction is to rub the area or put it under running cold water. While these cutaneous impulses are stimulated the pain diminishes. Electrical stimulation has the same effect and is the principle behind transcutaneous electric nerve stimulation (see Chapter 6), used as a method of pain control.

The gating mechanism can be affected by emotion and the impulses in the descending tracts from the brain stem, thalamus and cerebral cortex. Melzack and Casey (1968) found that the interaction of these systems and the evaluation of the pain input in terms of past experience provided perceptual information relating to the location, size and spatiotemporal properties of the noxious stimulus. These systems also provide a motivational tendency towards fight or flight, and cognitive information based on previous experience and the likely outcome of different strategies. The spinal cord acts as a centre for the integration and filtering of incoming sensory information.

Melzack and Wall found that there was another mechanism which operated in parallel with the gate-control and impulse-triggered mechanisms. When a peripheral nerve is cut, changes occur, altering the chemistry and physiology of the dorsal root ganglion cells, the motor neurones and the central terminals of the sensory fibres. Changes in afferent fibres produce a reduction in inhibition, a spread of receptive fields and increased excitability. These delayed peripheral and central changes are not produced by the nerve impulses. The time course and properties of the central changes support the theory that they are produced by changes in chemicals transported within the axons of sensory fibres. 'The complex sequences of behaviour that characterize pain are determined by sensory, motivational, and cognitive processes that act on motor mechanisms. By **motor mechanisms** Melzack and Casey mean all of the brain areas that contribute to overt behavioural response patterns.' (Melzack and Wall, 1991)

Summary

It is at the level of the dorsal horn that the first pain gate control comes into play. At its simplest, the theory states that within the spinal cord there are mechanisms that may open the gate to impulses generated by noxious (painful) stimuli so that we become aware of them – e.g. burning or knocking oneself. Other stimuli close the gate so that we become less aware of them – e.g. rubbing or shaking a limb to relieve pain. The gate control can be switched on by stress, exercise and intense stimulation. Chemicals, peptides and neurokinetics, are released when the nerve fibres are stimulated. The sympathetic nerve fibres release noradrenalin, acetylcholine and peptides, causing changes in the spinal cord which lead to an increase in excitability and nociceptive messages. The body produces its own morphine-like or pain-relieving chemicals. These substances are called endorphins and enkephalins and are found in areas of the brain and higher centres. The activation of pain receptors and ascending fibres by noxious stimuli activates the nociceptive or analgesic system via the opiate receptors which are found in the midbrain, medulla and dorsal horn areas of the CNS. Many areas of the brain send messages down to the spinal cord to help in the control of pain. One of these areas, the **limbic system**, gives an emotional 'charge' or 'weighting' to the individual's thinking, experience, memory and anticipation of pain. The other important mechanism in the control of pain is the endorphins and enkephalins which are released during exercise, relaxation and when the individual is feeling positive. From this it can be seen that pain can be affected in both a negative and positive way and that there are many factors involved in the control of pain.

The reader may find that some of the explanations of gate control theory are simplistic. For more detailed information read Chapter 10 of Melzack and Wall, 1991, Bowsher, 1986 and Melzack and Wall, 1965.

3

Pain concepts

THE MEDICAL MODEL

The medical model can be described as investigative, diagnostic (this usually means a physical or psychiatric diagnosis) and treatment-orientated. One diagnosis is expected and in all these interventions the doctor or therapist is the expert. The treatment is very 'cure'-orientated and the patient does not take an active part; they are passive recipients of treatment. Fordyce (1976) called this model the 'disease model perspective'. The essential features of this model were based on the assumption that the symptoms or indicators of pain were due to some process occurring within the individual. The doctor or health professional having identified these indicators, looks for the **cause** and then removes or reduces the cause by means of an action. If a physical cause cannot be found for the pain, then the symptoms may be identified as psychogenic or psychosomatic. That is, the pain symptoms are a consequence of a mental process. Fordyce referred to this model as a closed model because of its assumption that the cause is solely within the individual. This model is useful as a tool for measuring or investigating pain which is of recent onset and works well for acute pain but has little or no success with chronic pain.

THE CHRONIC PAIN MODEL

The chronic pain model illustrates the complexity of chronic pain. There are many problems associated with long-term pain. These may include physical debilitation, depression, side-effects of medication and dependence on family, friends and the medical profession. The individual may have suffered loss of job, loss of self-esteem and loss of role within the home environment and consequently their life is controlled by the pain. If the pain cannot be cured, other aspects of life such as regaining fitness, planning and achieving goals in life and reducing medication can be worked on. Working within this model the patients find that, although the pain may not improve, they are able to have control over their lives once again.

When the pain lasts for more than a few weeks other factors have to be taken into consideration, such as possible reinforcement of the pain and its consequent behaviours by the avoidance of activities that are difficult or distasteful to the individual. The evaluation of pain should include the identification of factors that maintain any pain behaviour, the influence of family relationships and the patient's role within the work, home and social situation. This model accepts that pain can be influenced by both internal and external processes and that it cannot be treated in isolation. It allows for both cognitive and behavioural aspects to be utilized in the treatment of an individual's pain.

MODEL OF PAIN MANAGEMENT

An increase in an individual's pain level can lead to a decrease in activity levels. This in turn leads to feelings of inadequacy and an inability to cope. People often say that they feel depressed or 'down'. They may also feel tense if they have a lot of pain and will say that they have experienced feelings of frustration and anger. The pain is influenced by both cognitive and behavioural factors: the individual modifies their activities in an effort to reduce the pain and this in turn leads to activities that the individual associates with pain being avoided.

Many factors are associated with pain; these can be split into three main categories: activities, thoughts and feelings (Figure 3.1).

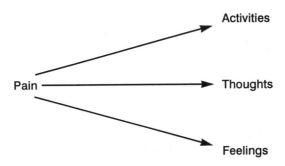

Figure 3.1 Pain cycle.

Pain cycle

Activities refers to any activity carried out in daily life such as washing, dressing, walking, hobbies or work-related activities. Thoughts about the inability to carry out tasks at work or in the home, about failing to fulfil a role, worries about finances or relationships and how people think about or see themselves are covered by the second category of thoughts. The third category of feelings covers the emotional aspects of pain, such as frustration, anger and achievement. It also refers to physiological aspects such as tension, sickness and fatigue.

Pain affects activity levels. If the individual is in a lot of pain, activity levels are likely to decrease. When this happens people often think about the difficulty of coping or holding down a job, and they feel tense, frustrated and angry at their inability to cope. However, the relationship between pain and activities, thoughts and feelings is a two-way process. The type of activity undertaken may well affect the level of pain experienced. For example if the individual walks further than usual, does too much housework or digs the garden for too long the pain level will increase. Patients commonly say that they 'pay later' when they increase their activity levels.

Pain patients tend to think or worry about their pain. At the back of their minds is the thought that the doctors might have missed something and this leads to them focusing on the pain. If they feel tense or unwell for reasons other than pain, for example a disagreement with family or illness, the pain level will tend to increase.

The three areas of activity, thoughts and feelings are not independent of each other: they are interrelated and cannot be considered in isolation. Unfortunately, this can lead to a vicious circle where the circle, and therefore the pain, can become self-sustaining (Figure 3.2).

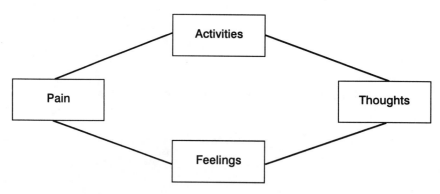

Figure 3.2   Vicious circle effect.

Most people with chronic pain have had their pain treated in the traditional model (medical model) with little or no effect. The individual presenting with chronic pain has proved that an approach based on 'curing' or affecting the pain will not work for them. However, activity, thoughts and feelings can be altered by teaching skills or coping strategies to achieve control in these three areas, thus eliminating the vicious circle effect and affecting the pain.

As can be seen from Figure 3.3 the arrows go both ways.

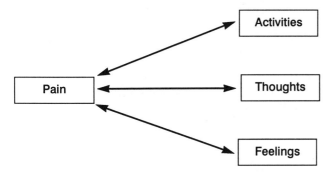

Figure 3.3   Two-way interaction in the pain cycle.

Pain affects activity levels, thoughts and feelings. However the reverse can also occur and activities, thoughts and feelings can affect the level of pain perceived by the individual. This model of pain management is based on the three systems model of emotions (Vlaeyen *et al.*, 1989), based on the fact that pain is frequently treated as a 'multifaceted condition involving gross motor, physiological and cognitive events' (Vlaeyen *et al.*, 1990).

Activity cycling

As discussed in Chapter 1 chronic pain leads to a change in people's activity levels. Many patients are not able to perform everyday tasks such as housework or cooking and they may need help with personal tasks such as dressing and bathing. Patients may have to be absent from work due to their pain and this in its turn reduces the individual's sense of self-worth and identity as a person. Many sufferers cope with their pain by spending much of the day resting and this can affect family and personal relationships. The commonest changes in activity or lifestyle are having to give up work due to pain, a reduced level of housework or social activity and a loss of role and self-esteem.

Underactivity/overactivity cycle

The patient often has a lifestyle that consists of periods of overactivity followed by resulting periods of underactivity. This leads to a routine of frequent rests during the day and avoidance of situations, people and activity that can cause stress or pain. The patient generally withdraws from social activity and their life becomes governed by the pain. They are often on high doses of medication, are drinking or smoking more and may have sleep problems. At this stage families and friends often report that they are a 'changed person'. Confronted with this downward spiral of reducing activity, long rest periods and increasing pain many patients suffer from depression and anxiety, which can result in broken relationships and loss of social contact.

This is a common cycle for people with chronic pain. The pain is the guiding factor and they tend to keep going until the pain tells them to stop. This is usually then followed by a period of rest, painkillers and feeling depressed and frustrated. People often say that 'the pain pays you back' or that 'you pay for it later!'

This cycle repeats itself time and time again (Figure 3.4). Each time it happens it reinforces the avoidance method of coping leading to reduced activity levels and increasing stiffness and weakness of the joints and muscles.

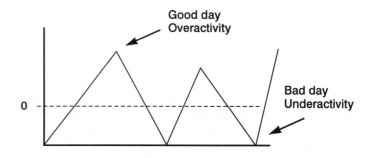

Figure 3.4   Overactivity/underactivity cycle.

The majority of people with chronic pain show this pattern, which is called **activity cycling**. In Figure 3.4, 0 represents a neutral point of activity. When the pain sufferer is having a 'good day', i.e. they are feeling positive, pain levels are reduced and they feel well in themselves. There is a tendency to increase the level of activity or output and because the individual feels 'well' this often results in overactivity. This can lead to a period of underactivity as the pain increases and is often accompanied by feelings of inadequacy due to the apparent failure to carry out normal activities or to maintain a normal lifestyle. With this continual overactivity/underactivity cycling there is never any real achievement or improvement in the pain condition: at best there is a maintenance of the status quo and at worst there is an overall reduction in activity and more frequent periods of inactivity. In the long term it is difficult to achieve any improvement because of this cycle of peaks and troughs.

To achieve change the peaks and troughs in activity need to be eliminated (Fig. 3.5). If the peaks of high activity can be avoided the troughs of low activity will gradually be eliminated making it much easier to undertake regular, steady levels of activity that can be maintained irrespective of the level of pain or discomfort.

Before the activity/pain cycle can be broken and activity levels can gradually be increased, the things that reinforce this type of behaviour should be identified. The three reinforcers are attention, rest and feedback. **Attention** should be given while activity is carried out and the person should be praised when they are successful. At the same time, disruptive behaviour should be ignored or paid little attention so that it is not reinforced. **Rest** should be introduced at regular planned intervals, following and during an activity, so that rest acts as a reinforcer and prevents the individual getting into the activity/pain cycle. **Feedback** should be given so that positive achievements are emphasized. Reinforcers are not the same for everyone and they should be used to gradually increase functional activity and minimize the pain caused by activity.

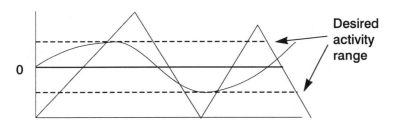

Figure 3.5   Reducing peaks and troughs of activity.

Chronic pain and lifestyle

People get into this vicious circle of overactivity/underactivity because when the pain is reduced there is a tendency to try and 'catch up' on all the things that have been left undone. Consequently there is a tendency to overdo things, with the result that the pain controls the level of activity. People tend to push themselves until the pain tells them to stop. The body starts to get out of condition, with joints becoming stiffer and muscles becoming weaker. Over a period of time the point at which the person achieves overactivity becomes lower and rest or low activity periods become longer, leading to a reduction in activity (Figure 3.6).

Positive aspects of activity cycling

Often there is work that has to be done today, it cannot be left for another day. If a job is finished and complete there is a sense of achievement. There is also an element of pleasure or enjoyment in carrying out some activities, especially a favourite hobby. In this situation the activity becomes engrossing and acts as a distraction from the pain. The individual may also be trying to ignore or 'beat' the pain by carrying out an activity.

Negative aspects of activity cycling

The negative consequences of activity cycling are that it may result in an exacerbation or flare-up of pain. There may be a temptation to avoid activities that cause pain and to take more rest periods, leading to a more inactive lifestyle. Over a period of time, activity cycling will lead to a reduction in activity levels. Pain will dictate the level of activity and consequently the individual becomes frustrated and depressed.

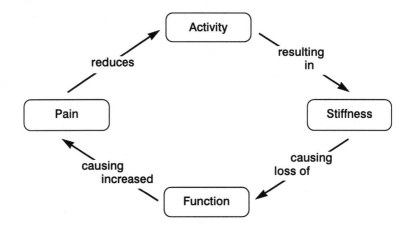

Figure 3.6   The affect of chronic pain on lifestyle.

RELATIONSHIPS AND ROLE

The chronic pain sufferer can be labelled as difficult, malingering and attention-seeking, by both their family and the medical profession. This exacerbates the problem, as the patient feels that no-one believes them, and their relationships within the family may suffer. They may take up an invalid role as their original role within the family is eroded away.

Other members of the family take over chores and may insist that the patient take it easy, forcing them into a passive role. Often activities which were once enjoyed are given up. The family may become overprotective so that the patient is unable to reassert their role within the family. Friends may fall away as the patient loses contact and has less interests in common with them (O'Hara, 1990).

Due to social isolation, loss of role and the inability to do things, people often get depressed. They can see no point in making plans and have nothing to look forward to. Depression often accompanies inactivity and creates a new set of problems. Often the person feels frustrated and a failure. This leads to a lack of motivation and desire to do things. Sleep may be disturbed, often leading to a reliance on sleeping tablets. Research has shown that depression increases the perception or feeling of pain.

With the cessation of normal activities, topics of conversation are reduced, depression causes lethargy and the pain causes the patient to become more irritable. Pain becomes the main focus of life and therefore of nearly all conversation and action. For the chronic pain patient, pain has taken over their life and gradually their social life, family and working life is affected and restricted by pain (O'Hara, 1990).

PAIN BEHAVIOURS

Pain behaviours are actions that the individual carries out when experiencing pain. For example, if they hit their finger with a hammer they may rub or hold the affected area, make facial grimaces and verbalize! The affected limb may even be nursed or cradled in an effort to protect it against further damage. These behaviours may be an immediate reaction to acute pain but when pain continues for a long time people often maintain such behaviours, usually subconsciously. Harvey (1988) found that the length of time the pain lasted influenced the amount of overt pain behaviour that was exhibited. Eventually the pain behaviours are elicited by external factors such as attention, sympathy and avoidance of unpleasant tasks. A study carried out by Fordyce, Caldwell and Hongadarin (1979) with a group of chronic pain patients found that pain behaviour in relation to exercise tolerance was not solely dependent on the experience of pain or the individual's perception of their pain. It could also be related to the length of time they had had the pain and other people's reaction to their pain behaviours.

People who have a long-standing pain problem often communicate pain through their behaviour. In this situation the pain behaviour may escalate in a subconscious effort to emphasize the reality of their pain. Often, patients come for assessment leaning heavily on a stick, wearing a collar or splint and displaying pain language or behaviour through posture and verbal utterances. Sometimes the patient may fall or stumble during assessment. Many of these behaviours are subconscious and occur because the patient is placed in a stressful situation with a consequent rise in body tension and individual stress levels. Many patients have been assessed in several departments before they reach the pain clinic or outpatient department where their condition is understood. In this situation pain behaviours are often more apparent, as the individual may feel that no one believes that they do have pain and that it must all be 'in the mind'. One of the things to be remembered when treating or assessing pain sufferers is that, however inappropriate the patient's behaviour, the pain is real to them. Whether it is stress factors that are feeding into the pain cycle, depression due to loss of role within the work and family situation or loss of self-esteem, the pain is real to the individual. When treating chronic pain patients the starting point for treatment is that the patient has pain.

Responses: behavioural, vocal and verbal

The nature of a person's psychological reaction to pain is determined by past experience and the degree of threat and frustration inherent in the pain. The most important factor affecting an individual's reaction to pain is the meaning the individual ascribes to it. If the person fears that the cause of the pain could be cancer, there may be a greater pain reaction until the biopsy is reported as negative.

Anxiety and depression can lower the pain threshold, increasing the patient's perception of pain. Anxiety may be related to the illness or treatment, to the anticipation of pain to come, or to other problems not related to the illness, such as work or home difficulties.

Reactions, as well as perceptions, are influenced by the amount of the patient's attention that is focused on the pain. If a situation requires concentration by the individual or creates pleasurable emotion, pain responses are minimized. The individual's responses to pain are also conditioned by social and cultural attitudes. Differences between groups of American women of different ethnic origins were studied by Sternbach and Tursky (1965) (Chapter 1). They found that women of Italian descent tolerated pain less well than those of Jewish or British descent. Zborowski (1969) also found that 'Anglo-Saxons' accepted their pain in a more matter-of-fact way and people of Mediterranean origin express their pain more readily. Although there were differences between the groups, these were ascribed to differences in culture rather than ethnic origin.

Beliefs and expectations can also determine the individual's reaction to pain. In East Africa an operation called 'trepanation' is carried out on men and women for the relief of pain. This operation is carried out without anaesthetics or drugs and involves cutting of the scalp and muscles to expose the skull, which is then scraped by the *doktari*. Films of this operation show the patients sitting calmly with no evidence of pain or discomfort (Melzack and Wall, 1991). The procedure is accepted as a method of chronic pain relief and it is the beliefs and expectations of this culture that influence the interpretation of the situation and technique as pain-free.

Previous pain experience can either increase or decrease the response to pain. Everyone has their own unique learning experience, which they bring to the situation, made up of those situations that have been observed and those that have been experienced. Zborowski found that the reactions of participants in his study on cultural influences were also closely allied to those observed within the family context in childhood.

The physical condition of a person can also affect the pain reaction or response. Fatigue and weakness can make pain seem less tolerable and the intensity and duration of the pain can make it difficult to cope with. Pain which has continued for a long time becomes tiring and may lead to over-reactive behaviour.

The emotional components of pain are interdependent with the physiological mechanisms of pain transmission and control. Both may aggravate the pain and increase the complexity and intensity of the response. Anxiety can result from pain and in turn anxiety may intensify it, resulting in a vicious circle. Physical and social functioning may be altered by the pain experience, leading to feelings of helplessness, isolation, fear and anxiety. Unless the cycle is interrupted these factors, singly or collectively, will continue to increase pain perception and intensity.

Chronic pain leads to endorphin depletion, which results in a lowering of the pain perception tolerance thresholds. Persistent pain may also cause loss of sleep and appetite, leading to general fatigue and disability. Uncontrolled pain frequently leads to disruptions in the family, social life and work. Physiological changes may lead to inefficient function and increased psychological responses to pain.

The behaviours which tell others that we have pain stop being 'effective' after a while, as other people get used to them. Most people with chronic pain recognize this and either they try to hide the fact that they are in pain or the behaviour that communicates pain becomes a permanent feature. Pain can be expressed through posture, facial and verbal expression. This in turn affects the reaction and behaviour of others towards the pain sufferer.

As their behaviour influences the response of others to them the pain-sufferer may need to ask themselves how they want to be treated – as a normal person or as someone who is disabled or sick? In asking this question the implications of the different behaviours or reactions have to be considered.

The advantages and disadvantages of normal behaviour

The advantages of normal behaviour are that the pain sufferer will not be treated differently, singled out or made to feel 'different'. Instead of being treated like an invalid the individual is able to interact with family and friends on a normal level.

The disadvantages of normal behaviour are that it is tiring to maintain the appearance of normality and the pain-sufferer may feel that they are carrying the burden of the pain alone and not getting any sympathy or understanding. Family and friends may also have a higher expectation of the individual's ability in relation to activity levels in the home and in the social and work environment.

The advantages and disadvantages of pain behaviour

The advantages of pain behaviour are that the pain sufferer will gain more sympathy and concessions in the form of assistance or consideration. The expectations of friends and family with regard to activity levels and social participation will be lower.

The disadvantages of pain behaviours are that they can become a habit even when the pain is not severe. Chronic pain sufferers often become absorbed in their pain and the effect it has on their lives. When this happens the only interest and topic of conversation may be the pain and its consequences. Friends react in various ways: by visiting less often, by avoiding questions about the individual's health and by not inviting the individual to participate in social events or activities. The majority of chronic pain sufferers want understanding, not sympathy.

Coping behaviours and perceived control

To minimize the impact of stressful situations or activities, people utilize coping strategies and Estlander and Harkpaa (1989) found that disability levels in pain patients were affected by the type of coping strategy used. One of the styles used is called **approach/avoidance coping**. People with approach coping skills confront the source of discomfort whereas people who utilize avoidance techniques avoid situations that may trigger it. Suls and Fletcher (1985) found that in a short-term, time-limited situation the avoidance coping strategy worked but in the long-term situation the approach coping strategy was more beneficial.

These findings were reinforced when Holmes and Stephenson (1990) carried out a study on the relationship between disability and coping in pain patients. They found that for acute pain situations avoidance copers had higher activity levels and in chronic pain situations activity levels were higher if the sufferer used approach coping strategies. In the acute pain situation the limb may be rested to enable healing to occur and the avoidance strategy is utilized effectively. However, if the avoidance situation is used in the chronic pain situation then the limb becomes stiff, range of movement decreases and pain increases. In chronic pain management the patient has to learn the approach coping strategy so that function and activity levels can be increased with a consequent decrease in stiffness, immobility and pain.

Perceived control is characterized in various ways such as 'locus of control', 'self-efficacy' or 'internal attribution'. Partridge and Johnston (1989) found that belief in control can predict disability levels following injury. Patients who believed that they had some control over their recovery had a lower disability level than those who did not. Fisher (1993) carried out a similar study where perceived control was changed (for a short while) and the resultant disability changes were monitored. Patients who were in the increased control conditions showed a reduction in disability and those in the decreased control condition had increased disability. **Self-efficacy** refers to the individual's expectations in relation to their ability to use pain reduction strategies effectively. Reese (1983) carried out a study that compared the effects of cognitive strategies, relaxation and pharmacological placebos on tolerance for pain using the cold pressor test. They were all equally effective in increasing the subject's expectation of pain relief. Bandura (1977) stated that self-efficacy is necessary but not sufficient for producing behavioural change. The higher the perception of self-efficacy in relation to a task the greater the likelihood of the individual initiating and persisting with that task. Other studies have observed that when pain-relief techniques are associated with positive self-efficacy this results in a greater reduction of the pain.

FAMILIES

The behaviour of other people affects a person's pain and how they communicate with them. Family and friends may be 'fed up' with the pain or may feel that it is best to ignore it and the behaviour that accompanies it. Others may be overprotective and sympathetic, constantly watching in case the person 'does too much' and encouraging them to rest so that the pain is not aggravated. They may prevent them from carrying out tasks by offering to do it for them. All these responses from family and friends are unhelpful in the long term, as they reinforce the invalid role of the sufferer and increase their feelings of failure and helplessness.

If the pain sufferer wants to change the family's attitude towards them they will first need to change their own behaviour. This in itself can create problems, as the family may not be able to cope with a more active positive person . They may be worried that a more positive approach on the part of the pain sufferer, with a consequence of increased activity levels, will result in an increase in pain.

COMMUNICATION

Communication has an important role to play in pain management. If family and friends understand what the person is trying to achieve they can work with them. When life has revolved around a person's pain it will take major adjustments, both for the pain sufferer and the family, to alter this. With long-term pain the individual's partner becomes tuned into the pain behaviours. Some will say things like 'I can tell from his/her face that the pain is worse'. In this situation the person tries to suppress pain behaviours until they are unable to do it any longer and then they manifest themselves in the form of an exaggerated response. This does not provide an answer to the problem in the long term. The pain sufferer needs to communicate clearly with family and friends with whom they interact closely and often. They need to explain what they are trying to achieve and the nature of their goals for managing pain.

For effective communication the pain sufferer has to be able to explain to their relatives, friends and doctor how their pain affects them. They need to be able to say 'No' when people's expectations of their abilities are unrealistic, and to explain why they are saying no. By being honest about their abilities communication is clearer and misunderstandings are avoided. Equally, the pain sufferer has to learn to ask for help or assistance when it is needed rather than suffering in silence or overdoing things – for example, asking the family to make their own beds or clear the table, or asking for help in packing bags and loading the car at the supermarket.

The type of communication used is important. It should not be aggressive or passive, it should be assertive. Assertive communication means being able to state clearly one's needs and intentions to other people so that they know how to respond. Pain sufferers find that the more clearly they can express themselves the more positive the response from others. Once the pain sufferer is able to acknowledge how a situation makes them feel (e.g. angry, frustrated, defensive), it often helps to let others know. However, this should be communicated calmly and assertively, not angrily or defensively in the heat of the moment.

Communication is a two-way process, which may consist of acknowledgement of the other person's viewpoint as well as the pain sufferer's own. In most situations there is room for compromise and negotiation. In acute or short-term pain most people are able to communicate or demonstrate to others that they have pain. However, with long-term pain these behaviours are in evidence all the time and people do not respond to them in the same way. Pain behaviours can affect the reaction of others to the pain sufferer. The first thing that is seen are the disability aids (stick, collar, splint), posture or expression and the initial reaction is to this and not the person behind the aids or behaviour.

Often, the pain sufferer will be given unwanted sympathy or may be treated as though it is 'all in the mind'. To be treated as a 'normal' person these behaviours need to be absent, so that the pain sufferer can be seen as an individual. Patients have to be prepared to challenge beliefs about what is good or bad for them, e.g. that people with back problems should not lift anything. It is not only the sufferer who needs to be re-educated, it is the families and partners as well.

4

Stress response

STRESS

Dr Benson (1976) defined stress as 'situations leading to continuous behavioural adjustment'. Everyone experiences stress at some time, whether it is when we oversleep and are late for work or the prospect of a visit to the dentist. Our perception of a stressful event is highly individual and is coloured by our previous experience and culture. Stress can be a positive as well as a negative force in our lives but if the stress continues for any length of time, the coping mechanisms of the individual may become ineffectual, resulting in increased anxiety, tension and fatigue.

History of stress theory

Descartes (1664) put forward the **psycho-physiological theory**, which proposed that emotions had a direct bearing on bodily responses. He saw the pineal body as the mediator between the sensory and motor functions and the soul, which experienced the emotions.

In 1935 Walter Cannon, the American physiologist, was one of the first people to use the term 'stress' in a non-engineering context. He saw stress as a disruption of the usual balance of a person's equilibrium. Cannon called this equilibrium or balance **homoeostasis**. Stress, in this context 'refers to those events or situations that challenge a person's psychological and/or physiological homoeostasis' (Carroll, 1992) The **Cannon–Bard theory** in the 1920s proposed a central mechanism for emotional reactions in the thalamus. It stated that the thalamus received sensory information and communicated with the cortex and bodily response systems, resulting in a behavioural response to the situation. This contradicted the **James–Lange theory** of the 1880s, which stated that bodily changes produced by the perception of an object or event could produce emotion.

General Adaptation syndrome

In the 1950s Hans Selye studied patients in hospital (Selye, 1956) and observed that, regardless of their illness or injury, they all exhibited the same patterns of physiological stress response. He called this the General Adaptation syndrome (GAS). The first stage is the alarm stage. This is an evaluative phase, where the threat or presence of the stressor is assessed. This results in increased levels of adrenocortical hormones in the body. The second stage is the resistance stage. At this stage the body tries to maintain normal functioning and adrenocortical hormone levels start to reduce. The final stage is the exhaustion stage, where the system becomes overloaded by the demands of the situation and people may exhibit symptoms of high blood pressure and stomach ulcers. From this we can see that, although the body is able to mobilize protective resources in an emergency, if the situation is prolonged resistance is lowered and when this occurs the individual is prone to infection. In chronic stress conditions there may be damage to the arteries due to a build up of cholesterol plaques, and increased acid levels in the stomach may result in ulcer formation. Selye's theory can be applied to psychological as well as physical stressors.

STRESS COMPONENTS

There are many types of stressor and everyone is different in the way they perceive them. Lazarus and Cohen (1977) suggested that there were three broad classes of stressors. They called them **cataclysmic events**, **personal stressors** and **daily hassles**.

Cataclysmic events

Cataclysmic events include natural disasters such as earthquakes and floods as well as man-made disasters such as wars. These can also be classified as **emergencies**. These events do not occur all the time, but when they do they can make us feel very stressed for a short time. They often affect whole communities and thus the stress effects may be counteracted by the mutual support and comfort provided within the community. The impact of this type of stress can be effectively counteracted by social support.

Personal stressors

The personal stressors, often called **negative life events**, include events such as losing one's job, divorce and death of a close relative. In the majority of cases the impact of these events is short-lived. The experience is individual rather than collective, unlike the cataclysmic events, in that different people have to face the experience at different times and therefore social support tends to be limited. There is evidence to show that negative life events are associated with physical illness. Research carried out by Rahe (1975) found that objective symptomatology and subjective ratings of illness showed a correlation to clusters of personal stressors. On the other hand, health may also be affected by the absence of positive life events. For example, in a study of 18-year-old Swedes, those who exhibited high blood pressure reported significantly fewer positive life events in the previous 2 years than those who were not hypertensive (Svensson and Theorell, 1983).

Daily hassles

Daily hassles are sometimes referred to as **background stressors**. They are chronic rather than acute stressors, and it is this that makes them serious. Daily hassles, like personal life events, are suffered by the individual. This type of stressor is continuous and is found in various areas such as work, driving, looking after children, money management and so on. A common source of daily hassle is the work environment. Carroll and Cross (1990) administered a battery of questionnaires to 1000 academic and academically related staff in seven British universities. Completed questionnaires were returned by 662 individuals and of these, 49% indicated that they found their jobs stressful either often or almost always. There was a high correlation between those reporting job stress and physical ill health.

RESPONSE TO STRESS

The stress response manifests itself in several ways both physically and psychologically. The body's physical reaction in the stress situation is often referred to as the 'fight or flight' response. When the stressor is experienced the autonomic part of the nervous system activates these responses, enabling action.

Physical response

The major somatic symptoms involve the tensing of muscles ready for movement, an increase in the breathing rate to supply the blood with plenty of oxygen and an increase in the heart rate to facilitate supplies of oxygen and other nutrients to the vital organs and muscles in the body.

Blood is directed away from the extremities (e.g. hands and feet) and the digestive system and is channelled to the brain and major muscles, where most of the activity is occurring or about to occur. The body also sweats more in order to cool this highly active system. People often complain of sweating palms and 'butterflies' in the stomach. Altogether there are about a dozen physical changes that occur, including hormonal and cardiovascular changes. This collection of responses is known as the **stress response**. It is the physical way the body responds to stress.

Psychological response

It is very important to try and identify the thoughts and feelings associated with stress. As well as the physical symptoms there may be feelings of anger, frustration, sadness, guilt and depression. People often say: 'Why me? I'm useless, I'm a failure, I can't do anything any more'. The psychological elements of the stress response are as important as the physical ones.

Psychological stress can manifest itself in various ways. A high level of anxiety and frustration can cause an increase in muscle tension, especially around the neck and shoulders. The tensing of muscles in response to a stressful situation can become a habit and eventually the level of tension in the neck and shoulders, or other areas of the body, becomes higher. The baseline for relaxation of the muscles becomes higher and the general level of tension in the muscles at relaxation is raised. When this happens secondary symptoms such as tension headaches, a tight chest or low back pain may occur. When pain is constant this can cause stress, as it is accompanied by feelings of tiredness and general debility.

Role of perception

'Perception refers to the means by which information acquired from the environment via the sense organs is transformed into experiences of objects, events, sounds, etc.' (Roth and Frisby, 1989). For example, a mouse might run across the floor. Some people's stress response would be activated by this because they are afraid of mice. Others would not react at all. However, they all see the same mouse; the difference is in how it is perceived – either as something to be feared because it poses a threat or as a non-threatening occurrence. Thoughts have a key role in stress and its management. Thoughts influence the body's reaction to stress.

Lazarus *et al.* (1965) found that altering a person's perception of a stressful event by the use of denial or intellectualization of instructions prior to the watching of the event lowered the person's perceived stress. Freud referred to these psychological mechanisms for reducing the impact of stress as **defence mechanisms** or **coping strategies**. Some individuals are more skilled than others in utilizing coping strategies and this may in part be a result of their previous life experience, genetic makeup and cultural influences. The perception of any situation is coloured by experience and how others behave or react in similar situations.

Feelings

Certain situations will produce specific emotions or feelings. For example, when someone is let down this can result in feelings of sadness, anger or frustration, whereas achieving a personal goal can make the individual feel happy, successful and positive about tackling any future goals. Long-term health problems, such as chronic pain, produce a whole range of feelings (both positive and negative) as people learn to cope with the frustrations, disappointments and readjustments that these problems incur.

Feelings and emotions in turn produce certain types of thinking. Frustration, anger and disappointment lead to negative thoughts. These thoughts are very destructive and can place extra pressure on the pain sufferer. Negative thinking can also block positive action. Negative thoughts create a vicious circle, which prevents the pain sufferer from taking positive action. This feeds into the negative feelings or emotions and proves the negative thoughts to be true. It becomes a self-fulfilling prophecy.

Positive thinking leads to positive action. Thinking positively and taking positive steps to cope with problems or situations can increase the individual's self-esteem. Thinking is the most important part of the stress response. Like the physical part of the stress response, the type of thinking that triggers it can become a habit.

Often the sources of stress are specific worries or thoughts, and they can act as a trigger. For example if driving is a stressful experience, thinking about the journey may trigger the stress response before even getting into the car. It is important for the pain sufferer to try and identify the thoughts and feelings associated with stress. Negative thoughts are intrusive and need to be challenged and replaced with positive thoughts.

THE HABITUAL AND CUMULATIVE NATURE OF STRESS

The stress response which occurs in the 'fight or flight' situation can also be produced by the body in response to non-emergency stressors. If this stress response is continually reproduced in non-emergency situations, it becomes the normal response to everyday events – it becomes a **habit**. This is a gradual process, resulting in a build-up of muscle tension, increased heart rate and breathing rate. As this process is acting at the level of the subconscious it creates a problem. Most people do not recognize the increase in physical tension until they reach point 'X' on Figure 4.1.

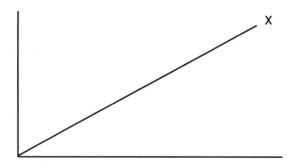

Figure 4.1 Cumulative stress response.

This is the point at which the body starts to produce secondary symptoms that reflect the fact that it is under stress. For example, people recognize that they are feeling stressed or tense because they experience a variety of symptoms. These may include tension headaches, low back pain, a tight feeling in the chest or problems with breathing. At this stage the stress response has become a habit and in some people may manifest itself as a panic attack, resulting in avoidance of situations that trigger the feelings.

DISEASE MODEL

As discussed earlier, the disease model (Fordyce, 1976) assumes that the indicators of pain, i.e. the symptoms of the patient, are a result of some process lying within the person. The doctor identifies the presence of symptoms indicating a pain problem, looks for the cause of the symptoms and then takes action to eliminate or minimize the cause (Fordyce, 1984). There is a constant seeking for the cause of the pain, which by default has to be treatable. If a physical cause cannot be found then the pain is assumed to be in the mind. This may be referred to as **psychogenic** or **psychosomatic manifestation**. Other labels are hysteria, hypochondriasis, personality problem and malingering. The common feature of all these terms is the inference that the pain symptoms are occurring as a consequence of some mental process.

BEHAVIOURAL MODEL

Clinical pain, when seen from the perspective of a behavioural or learning/conditioning model may result in different inferences from the disease model. These differences are relevant to the understanding, diagnosing and managing of clinical pain. Pain problems are often manifested by the behaviour of the patient. Without visible or audible indications from the patient of their pain, there may be no indication of a problem. Behaviours of patients that indicate the presence of pain are pain behaviours and may be appropriate or inappropriate. Because they are behaviours they are subject to the same factors as influence our everyday behaviour. The behavioural model can be seen as an open system. Events that are critical to the occurrence/non-occurrence of pain behaviours may be external to the person in the present or future environment.

The essential element of behavioural strategies for enabling change to occur is helping the patient to develop alternative behaviours or strategies. In the context of treating chronic pain, this consists of re-establishment of their role within the work and family situation, and raising of self-esteem and feeling of worth. The patient needs to feel in control of the situation, instead of feeling that the situation is controlling them. There are various procedures which can be used and the essential point is to recognize that helping a person to reduce or

eliminate a behaviour is of no use unless it is replaced by a workable alternative. For example, it is easier to help a patient increase their standing and walking tolerance times than to decrease the time they spend lying down because of
the pain. Patients and their families need to be fully involved in the process, and
discussion and explanation of the treatment process must be fully participative.

STRESS MANAGEMENT

Stress management is an important part of pain management. In addition to all
the normal stresses and strains of everyday life the pain sufferer has the addi-
tional problem of coping with ill health. 'Stress in scientific terms is the wear
and tear induced in the body by the adaptive day to day struggle of the organism
to remain normal in the face of potentially harmful agents, including physical
and psychological stressors of all kinds, from bad food to noisy neighbours'
(Mackarness, 1976).

Knowing the source of the stress does not, in itself, help the individual to
cope with it when it occurs. Although such sources can be avoided and lifestyle
can be modified, the individual must first learn how to recognize and deal with
the signs and effects of stress.

Cluster theory

It is not only the unpleasant things of life that act as stressors, it is also events
that are planned for and looked forward to, such as holidays and weddings.
There are few events that do not have some accompanying stress element.
Psychiatrists at the University of Washington Medical School gave a list of 43
commonly occurring events in human life to 394 men and women of varying
ages and social backgrounds and asked them to rate the events mathematically
for their stress impact, with the most stressful rating 100 'life change units'. As
a fixed point to work from, they were told that a marriage was assessed at 50
units. The basis of judgement was the effort of adjustment acquired in living
through an event. The list was called the **Social Readjustment Rating Scale**.
When averages were calculated, the death of a spouse was ranked at the maximum 100 life change units. In follow-up studies they found that 10 times more
widows and widowers died during the 12 months following the death of a
husband or wife than all other people in their age groups. It was also found that
illness was 12 times more likely during the year following divorce than in
married persons during a corresponding year.

When several life change events on the inventory come together or 'cluster',
people are more susceptible to illness and this occurs in the months following
the period of stress rather than during it. However, the impact of life change
events varies according to the temperament and conditioning of the individual
and the event's circumstances. It was also found that when life change events
are welcomed the stress impact is greatly reduced.

STRESS-RELATED DISORDERS

Stress is seen as a contributory factor in cardiovascular disorders, immunological disorders and upper respiratory problems. Many of these disorders have been found to have a direct relationship to stress which is work-related or to situations where the individual perceives themselves to be lacking in social support.

Executive stress

'Executive stress' is one of the cliche terms of our times, linked with an image of a harassed businessman wincing at a stab of pain from a stomach ulcer. However, research has shown that being unemployed can be even more stressful than having a responsible job and a significant increase in illness and premature deaths is linked with unemployment. People who are unemployed become frustrated and depressed. The consequences of this situation in a climate of redundancies and low job availability are that the individual may have financial worries and feel inadequate, and that their role within the family has been eroded because they are no longer the bread-winner. If the situation continues over a protracted time span they may start to feel that they don't have support from their family, as other family members may take over the role of wage-earner. They may also lose structure and meaning in their life and say that there is no reason to get up in the morning and that there is nothing to look forward to. In this situation stress levels are raised and the individual may become anxious and depressed and as a consequence more susceptible to viral infections and diseases.

Studies carried out in Europe and the USA show the influence of occupation on the incidence of high blood pressure, heart disease, duodenal ulcers and diabetes among the workforce. These disorders were prevalent among workers who had a high level of responsibility. A study carried out on American air traffic controllers, who worked for long periods in a state of high alertness, found a higher incidence of hypertension, duodenal ulcers and diabetes than in pilots (Carroll, 1992). The problem for workers in high responsibility and peak alertness jobs is to 'unwind' after the day's work.

Heart disease

The most prevalent diseases associated with stress are high blood pressure and heart problems. Several factors are responsible for the prevalence of these disorders in developed countries. A high level of saturated animal fats in the diet is much debated as a factor, as is insufficient exercise and stress. Statistical evidence has linked stressful living with high blood pressure. In the United States more black than white people suffer from high blood pressure, but this only applies to black people who live in the urban ghettos not to those in rural areas, and the incidence is halved in the middle-class suburbs of cities.

A stressful emotion can cause a build-up in the blood of fatty substances, such as cholesterol and triglycerides, which may stick to the walls of the arteries, causing narrowing. During an alarm or stress response cortisone levels in the blood go up, and high cortisone levels have been known to damage heart tissue.

Friedman *et al.* (1986) carried out a study on the personality traits and lifestyles of people with heart disease. They found that there were two contrasting behaviour types: one prone to coronary disease and one with a high chance of avoiding it. The first group, type A, was ambitious, aggressive, impatient, self-demanding and always in a hurry. The second group, type B, was less rushed, less ambitious, had a more philosophical perspective on things, was rarely impatient and was able to enjoy the present. The first group, who suffered from continual psychological stress, were more prone to heart disease.

Some studies have suggested that stress weakens the body's defences against infection and that the capacity of the immune system to destroy bacteria is impaired when there is an excess of stress-response steroids in the blood. Studies carried out in people who were recently divorced or separated found that there was a higher incidence of ill health compared with a group who were married, widowed or single. Research has shown that marital disruption can be a predictor of physical illness.

Arnetz *et al.* (1987) looked at the impact of unemployment on the individual. They concluded that loss of time structure during the day, social contact, achievement, collective goals, identity, social status and activity all contributed to the individual's increased stress and anxiety levels, low self-esteem and susceptibility to ill health. When blood tests were taken there was evidence of reduced reactivity in the immune system.

Other researchers have shown that an excess of adrenaline in the blood slows down the repair of tissue and the renewal of cells. Tension keeps adrenaline at high levels in the blood, whereas the output of adrenaline is reduced during relaxation or sleep, promoting repair and renewal in the body. Relaxation has been found to promote the healing of skin cuts and wounds, and tension to retard healing. Stress management training and techniques, such as relaxation, have also been shown to reduce high blood pressure.

Upper respiratory tract disorders

House *et al.* (1979) looked at factors that made the individual more likely to seek medical advice for symptoms of illness. They found that there was a positive association between reports of stress at work and complaints of physical symptoms such as upper respiratory tract infections and coughs. This association was only reliable for subjective reporting of the disorder and did not necessarily coincide with actual medical evidence. Work is a source of stress because there may be conflicting or excessive demands placed on the individual in the workplace. This may be due to staff shortages, sickness or unrealistic deadlines and this type of stress is no longer reserved for the business executive.

Immunological disorders

Stress is said to increase the risk of infectious diseases such as influenza and colds. However the implication that stress plays a causal role in these disorders has been disputed because much of the research has involved retrospective analysis of life events in the period preceding the infection. Although stress and depression are associated with a reduction in activity of the immune system this does not mean that stress makes the individual more susceptible to infection. Stress may cause alterations in an individual's behaviour, which may result in a poor diet, increased smoking or alcohol intake and lack of exercise and sleep. These in turn may make the individual more prone to infection.

Effects of perceived control and support

Alfredsson, Spetz and Theorell (1985) carried out a study on the deaths of people from heart disease. They found that it was commonest amongst workers who had least control over their work, what they did and when they did it. Theorell et al. (1985) also found an association between occupational demand, control by the worker and objective health indicators. More recent studies have shown that control of a situation is a crucial factor in the determination of the effect of a given stressor. Studies of the elderly in residential homes have found that they are healthier if they have an input to the running of the home; this may involve tasks such as laying of tables at mealtimes, helping in the greenhouse or planning social events. A potentially stressful situation in the workplace may become a challenge if the individual perceives that they have some control over the way the work is carried out. A situation where there is no apparent control, for example sitting in a queue of traffic on the motorway, can be stressful but if the individual can ring their home or workplace to let them know about the delay the stress is reduced, as they have regained control of the situation. Glass and Singer (1972) found that the impact of stress is reduced if the individual perceives that they are in control.

There is also evidence to suggest that social support can counteract the effects of stress. In this context 'social support' 'refers to the provision of comfort, caring, esteem, or help by other people or social groups' (Carroll, 1992). A study carried out by Brown and Harris (1978) among 400 women living in South London found that some women were more prone to depression following stressful events. There were several predisposing factors but the main one was the absence of a close and supportive relationship. In a study on the risk of coronary disease, Orth-Gomer and Unden (1990) found that low levels of social support could predict death from coronary heart disease. Research on recovery from coronary episodes showed that psychological stress exacerbated symptoms whereas social support had the opposite effect (Fontana et al., 1989).

Assessment

5

FACTORS TO CONSIDER WHEN ASSESSING

Creek (1990) said that assessment is 'the measurement of the quality or degree of the various factors in a situation or condition'. Assessment is essential for diagnosis and the planning of pain control and other therapeutic treatment. The assessment process should enable the therapist to gain an understanding of the patient's pain and how it affects their activity levels in the home, at work and in the social situation. It should also identify the factors that ease or aggravate the pain, at what time of day it is at its worst and whether it is constant or intermittent. It is necessary to ascertain from the patient details of any medication, how it is taken and whether it is taken on a regular basis or only when the pain is unbearable. The assessment should cover the previous medical history and details of any other treatment currently being received or undertaken. The present family situation and any help received should also be documented. This information will help the therapist to gain a picture of the patient's medical and social profile and enable them to formulate a treatment programme with the patient to facilitate control of the pain. Choiniere *et al.* (1990) consider that accurate assessment will enable the medical team to monitor the patient's progress, evaluate the effectiveness of medication or treatment and make an accurate diagnosis. If there is no physiological method of pain assessment then the therapist is reliant on the verbal report of the patient.

Various assessment tools are available; they vary in content, structure and complexity. In choosing the most suitable tool for assessment the following aims should be met.

- The tool should enable the therapist to ascertain the duration, intensity and quality of the pain. This in turn should aid diagnosis and act as an indicator for therapy.
- The assessment should act as an evaluation mechanism for the treatment or therapy chosen.
- The patient's age, physical and psychological status, and the level of comprehension and compliance they are capable of will influence the pain assessment tool used.

- Other influences are the time available for administration, the expertise of the staff and ease of use of the chosen assessment tool.

Assessment has a subjective element as the therapist is unable to feel the patient's pain but may empathize or use their own experience to try and understand or evaluate it.

PAIN IS SUBJECTIVE

Pain is difficult to measure because it is subjective. Only the person experiencing the pain knows how it feels, its intensity, location and the restrictions it places on their lives. However, assessment is needed for diagnosis and planning of its treatment and control. 'Pain is whatever the experiencing person says it is, existing whenever the experiencing person says it does' (McCaffery and Beebe, 1989). This definition is the starting point for any assessment of a person with pain problems. The patient's distress, caused by the pain, also distresses the family and they should be involved in any treatment or management offered. They can form a valuable support network for the patient while treatment is in progress. As pain is a subjective process the assessor must learn to recognize 'pain cues' and to evaluate the severity of the pain as objectively as possible.

Beliefs and values

One of the problems is that both the doctor and the patient have values and beliefs relating to the pain response and how it is reported. These beliefs and values may differ. When examining the patient the doctor may find that the patient has a good range of movement and no apparent restriction, although the patient is complaining of pain. The patient may not be a good communicator, or it may be that the pain is only there when carrying out a specific activity, e.g. sitting or standing for long periods. Because someone does not look as though they are in pain or does not have any objective signs it does not necessarily follow that there is no pain. Lavies et al. (1992) and Zalon (1993) found that pain could be both under- and overestimated, causing bias.

In the evaluation of pain it is important to distinguish between bias and inaccuracy. Other studies, carried out with doctors and nurses, illustrate that health professionals may find it difficult to assess pain accurately and to estimate the degree of pain experienced by the patient (Sutherland et al., 1988; Choiniere et al., 1990). Such inaccuracy can be overcome by training staff in the use of the evaluation tools available and ensuring that recorded observations are within agreed guidelines or set criteria. Bias can be minimized by encouraging patient participation when filling in charts or analogue scales so that the pain rating is quantified by their perception rather than that of the professional.

The Royal College of Surgeons of England (1990) states that 'systematic pain assessment is essential if pain is to be managed effectively'. Mather and Mackie (1983) found that children played down their pain because they did not want to be given an injection. In this instance the children were capable of evaluating their pain and using the visual analogue scale available to do this. However, the consequences of accurate reporting were unpleasant and so the pain report was inaccurate. Similarly, adult patients will minimize their pain report and will suffer in silence because they do not want to be a burden or a 'nuisance' to the nursing staff or their family.

Patients' beliefs about their pain often influence their pain experience. Schwartz, DeGood and Shutty (1985) assessed pain beliefs by getting the patients to view an educational videotape on pain clinics and the techniques used in pain management. Some patients rated the video as applicable to their own beliefs and others that it was irrelevant to their pain. The results of a later study indicated that those patients who found the tape irrelevant had higher levels of pain, lower levels of physical activity and were dissatisfied with treatment (Shutty, DeGood and Hoekstra, 1987). In 1989 Williams and Thorn developed the Pain Beliefs and Perceptions Inventory. They found that those patients who said that they expected their pain to persist showed poor compliance with physical therapy and behavioural interventions. Patients who had lower levels of pain were those who blamed themselves for their pain.

ADAPTATION TO PAIN

Patients can adapt to pain both behaviourally (by restricting their activities) and physiologically. This can manifest itself as periods of minimal pain or the person showing no obvious signs that they are in pain. Physiologically the body tries to maintain its equilibrium. If the body's initial response to pain was maintained for long periods there would be permanent physical damage and so the body returns to normal for a while so that equilibrium can be restored. Behaviourally the body can become accustomed to a level of pain and if this continues for any length of time the body takes up postures or behaviours to cope with it.

Illness and pain are fatiguing, and some patients may react by being quieter than usual and by lying or sitting still because they are too tired to do anything else. Patients sleep because the body is exhausted but this does not mean that while they sleep they are pain-free. While the patient is sleeping or resting the body can conserve energy. Others may show little response to pain because they have devised their own coping strategies. They may have found that reading, carrying out a hobby that absorbs them, listening to music or watching television acts as a distraction from the pain. Some patients simply put on a 'brave face' and do not show that they are in pain. This can be a cultural response or influenced by the individual's upbringing and family background.

Research carried out on pain in childbirth found that many factors influenced the severity of the pain experienced. If the mother was unhappy about the birth, had little support from family and friends and was afraid of coping with the pain associated with the birth then the pain level was increased (Read and Cox, 1985; Fridh *et al.*, 1988). Conversely, mothers who had already experienced a lot of pain unrelated to childbirth reported less painful deliveries (Niven and Gijsbers, 1984). Bonnel and Boureau (1985) also found that the level of discomfort or pain displayed was different according to the cultural background of the woman. Research has shown that behavioural and physiological signs are not reliable as indicators of pain severity. Houde (1982) considered that a patient's self-report was the most accurate way to quantify pain.

Pain perception

The duration and intensity of a pain stimulus will vary between individuals. In the medical profession there is an expectation of an individual's response following certain procedures – i.e. the level of pain, its intensity and its duration. These expectations are only guidelines and cannot be taken as absolute definitions of the individual's likely response. Melzack *et al.* (1987) carried out a study of patients post-surgically. They found that 31% had pain beyond the fourth day due to complications. They received inadequate analgesia, as the staff's expectations of the intensity of the pain were not the same as the patient's actual pain. This reinforces the fact that the duration and intensity of pain are variable between individuals with comparable conditions.

These findings are supported by the gate control theory, which maintains that there are different factors that can influence the closing of the gate. It can be partially closed if the large fibres are stimulated by rubbing, and inhibition of the pain impulses may come from the brain stem due to sensory input via distraction. Inhibition may also come from the cortex because the patient's experience of pain indicates that it will be short-lived. Studies have shown that the perceived level of pain is greater if there is no inhibition.

In 1985 an epidemiological study was carried out nationally. The results indicated that there was a high prevalence of pain in the general population. It was also found that women and those people whose parents had suffered pain were more likely to experience some form of pain, e.g. backache, muscle or joint pain (Taylor and Curran, 1985).

Pain tolerance and thresholds

Each individual has their own unique response to pain. Pain tolerance 'is the intensity of pain that an individual is willing to accept without seeking pain relief' (Sofaer, 1992). Sometimes people are said to have a **low pain tolerance**, i.e. their ability to cope with pain is low. This may be affected by psychological and cultural factors, current anxiety level and past experience. In general, physiological signs and behaviours are easier to observe when assessing pain than the patient's own verbal report. Factors that should be taken into account are the individual's subjective report of the pain and everything that influences it. For example, in childbirth women may tolerate high pain levels without medication because they want to be alert for the delivery, or because they are worried that medication might harm the baby.

Often, pain tolerance is influenced by the expectations of family and friends. Mild pain is usually tolerated for longer than pain which is severe. However if the pain is prolonged or recurrent then this will lower the individual's pain tolerance level. In many cultures pain tolerance is seen as an indicator of maturity and in primitive tribes there are often associated rites to mark this passage of development in the adolescent's life. Pain thresholds are affected by factors such as anxiety and stress. In various clinical conditions, such as osteoarthritis of the hip, the threshold can alter but once the pain is relieved the threshold returns to normal.

ASSESSMENT OF PAIN

Pain can be measured both subjectively and objectively to assess the effects of treatment and any fluctuations in pain severity. The sensory and emotional aspects of pain cannot be measured directly and are both subjective and individual to the sufferer. The autonomic and motor components of pain can be measured more objectively. Measurements of the pain threshold, discrimination and pain tolerance may be used. The **pain threshold** refers to the least amount of stimulus required to produce a sensation or response. **Discrimination** refers to the smallest change in stimulus intensity that can be detected and **pain tolerance** refers to the point at which the subject is forced to withdraw from the stimulus.

Acute pain assessment

If the patient has not had a thorough investigation of their pain problem the consultant may request blood tests, X-rays or scans. The patient may be then be referred to the appropriate speciality for further treatment or a second opinion. Physical assessments may include the assessment of pain at rest and on movement and, for surgical patients, pain on coughing. Patients awaiting hip replacement may have increased pain levels when getting dressed, getting out of a chair or walking. Pain should be assessed pre- and post-surgery for an accurate evaluation of pain relief. Any intervention that gives pain relief should be assessed on a regular basis and pain assessment should include the level of distress caused to the individual. Wherever possible the patient should be actively involved in the assessment. If other symptoms such as nausea, vomiting, or sedation are associated with the pain or its treatment these should also be reported and assessed.

Chronic pain assessment

Patients who are referred to a chronic pain group usually present having tried many avenues of treatment, both medical and complementary, none of which appear to have helped. Often the patient reports that they were worse following the treatment. The original cause of the pain has been treated, but the patient still complains of feeling pain and finds that it is taking over their life. With the more chronic patient the pain controls their lives, they suffer from low self-esteem and loss of role within the home and workplace. When the patient is examined in the initial assessment the consultant will note any inappropriate signs and symptoms, e.g. exaggerated reaction to light touch, groans, facial grimaces and holding of the limb or painful area of the body. The consultant also looks at the type of pain, initial causation and whether it can be controlled or treated by medication, or possibly an injection into the painful site as in scar pain and trigger point pain. If the patient is suffering from an orthopaedic problem, such as a back or neck problem, the appropriate physical examination is carried out.

Physical assessment

The assessment of patients with pain problems can be divided into several areas. The consultant will conduct a physical examination to determine whether the pain has an obvious cause and, if so, whether it can be treated by conventional methods such as physiotherapy, medication or injections, or whether surgery is appropriate. The consultant will also consider whether the type of pain and its location indicate that there is a physical cause such as nerve root entrapment or a disc lesion causing pressure on the nerve. Thirdly, an assessment will be made as to whether the patient has signs of anxiety or depression and is exhibiting pain behaviour. The patient's ability to carry out tasks independently – e.g. getting in and out of a chair, on and off the bed – the way they walk and generally use or hold the body will be considered. Finally, the consultant will decide whether the patient needs to have further investigations, be referred for a second opinion or be seen by another specialist.

WADDELL'S THEORY

Gordon Waddell, Professor of Orthopaedic Surgery in Glasgow, carried out some studies in the 1980s (Waddell *et al.*, 1984) on a patient's suitability for spinal surgery. His studies found that the number of inappropriate signs and symptoms that the patient presented with, in the clinical situation, could be a contraindication for surgery. Patients who presented with several of these inappropriate signs and symptoms did not have a good recovery postoperatively, and often the pain was worse or more debilitating. Some had an initial good result but then became worse again. Waddell (1984) said that the signs and symptoms of illness behaviour were 'observable and potentially measurable actions and conduct which express and communicate the individual's own perception of disturbed health'. The patient is assessed in the following ways, by **observation**, **physical examination** and the noting of any **chronic illness behaviour** (Table 5.1).

Table 5.1   Observation and physical examination

Assessment	Aspect assessed	Range covered
Observation	Posture/rhythm/flexion/ extension/lateral flexion/gait	Standing/walking
Physical examination	Range of movement	Carried out in supine/prone/ sitting/standing positions
	Check for abnormal neurology signs	
	Check for nerve root entrapment	
	Check reflexes	
	Other investigations	Blood test/X-ray/MRI/ radiculogram

Observation

The Consultant observes whether the posture, rhythm of movement and the walking gait of the patient are normal or abnormal; whether flexion, extension and lateral flexion are normal or limited; and whether simulated rotation produces pain.

Physical examination

During the physical examination the consultant checks the range of movement in the spine, legs and hips, also that there are no abnormal neurology signs and that there is no evidence of nerve root entrapment. This examination is carried out standing, lying in the supine and prone positions and sitting. Depending on the diagnosis the consultant may also wish to see the patient walking across the room. The patient's reflexes, i.e. ankle and knee jerk reflex, are checked. The consultant may carry out further investigations to eliminate disorders such as rheumatoid arthritis or osteoarthritis. Other investigations may include blood tests, X-rays, MRI scans and radiculograms.

Chronic illness behaviour

Table 5.2 lists the criteria Waddell formulated for assessment of illness behaviour; many orthopaedic surgeons and pain consultants use them in their routine examinations of patients with back problems. The criteria can also be observed in other pain disorders.

Table 5.2   Signs and symptoms of illness behaviour

	Physical disease	*Illness behaviour*
Symptoms		
Pain	Localized	Tailbone
		Whole leg
Numbness	Dermatomal	Whole leg numb
Weakness	Myatomal	Whole leg gives way
Time pattern	Episodic	Never pain-free
Treatment response	Variable benefit	Never successful
		Emergency admissions
Signs		
Simulated rotation	No pain	Non-anatomical pain
Axial loading	No pain	Pain
Straight leg raising	Same on distraction	Improves on distraction
Sensory	Dermatomal	Regional
Motor	Myatomal	Regional
General reaction	Appropriate	Over-reaction

The symptoms of illness behaviour

Pain is not localized: the patient may complain that the pain is in the tailbone or in the whole leg. The distribution of **sensation loss** is not dermatomal: the patient complains of the whole leg feeling numb. Any **weakness** of the limb has a distribution that is not myatomal and the patient may complain of the whole leg giving way. The **time pattern** is not episodic and patients tend to report that they are never pain-free.

   Response to treatment is variable, but if the patient is exhibiting illness behaviour they will often say that none of the treatments have helped. Patients have often had several emergency admissions to the hospital with their pain problem.

The signs of illness behaviour

Tenderness is not localized, it is superficial, widespread and non-anatomical. The patient often complains of tenderness and pain in response to light touch. If **rotation** is simulated, i.e. the arms are held to the side and the whole body is turned from side to side, the patient complains of pain. If **axial loading** is applied the patient complains of pain (this is carried out by putting pressure on the shoulders or the head). In **straight leg raising** the pain improves on distraction. Where pain is caused by physical disease there is no difference when the patient is distracted.

Sensory loss is regional in distribution rather than dermatomal and **motor loss** is regional in distribution rather than myatomal. The **general reaction** of the patient is that of over-reaction to examination, i.e. they respond inappropriately. Often the patient groans while carrying out a movement, holds the painful area, grimaces or has abnormal postures in sitting, standing and walking.

Although pain has a protective purpose in signalling tissue damage, when the pain continues for a length of time this may no longer be the case. In the chronic situation the patient may have an abnormal or over-reaction to pain. If the patient has had the pain for some time, reactions may be learned. For example, if a particular activity or situation increases or triggers the pain the patient will start to avoid this activity or situation. If it cannot be avoided then the patient may take up abnormal postures or brace the body to try and counteract the pain. Eventually this response is triggered as soon as the activity or situation is encountered, i.e. before the body has time to register pain. It becomes a learned behaviour.

Chronic illness behaviour does not mean that the patient is not feeling pain: their reaction to the situation has been shaped or moulded by experience. In the same way, by verbalizing their pain or limping or holding the painful area they elicit sympathy and concern from relatives and friends, thus reinforcing the behaviour. The patient often gets into the vicious circle of activity, pain, rest, stiffness and pain, activity, and so on. These peaks and troughs of activity and pain are self-sustaining, and the chronic patient is often unable to break the cycle without help. A group programme may be beneficial to this category of patient. Fordyce (1976) stated that 'because pain behaviours are overt they are particularly susceptible to conditioning and learning influences' (Keefe and Williams, 1989). A series of studies carried out by Keefe and Block (1982) found that motor pain behaviours could be observed and used as a valid index of pain.

ASSESSMENT TOOLS

There are a number of pain assessment tools in the literature (Melzack, 1987; McCaffery and Beebe, 1989) and there is evidence to suggest that consistent use of these tools does help with the control and management of pain. There appear to be three main types used, categorical scales (CAT), visual analogue scales (VAS) and the McGill Pain Questionnaire (MPQ).

Pain charts and diaries

Categorical scales are often incorporated into pain charts and diaries. These verbal rating scales are used to measure pain relief and pain intensity. Categories vary from 4 to 10. The higher the number of categories the more sensitive the scale. McQuay (1990) found that there was a tendency for pain intensity scales to be less sensitive than pain relief scales. This type of scale is often used because it has been found to be reliable and consistent (Jensen, Karoly and Braver, 1986), it correlates well with the VAS (Max, Portonoy and Laska, 1991) and it is quick and easy to use.

The pain charts and diaries (Table 5.3) are filled in by the patient or nurse.

Table 5.3 Example of daily diary – pain amount would be scored on a scale of 0–10 and mood on a similar scale ranging from not depressed to extremely depressed; patients may enter use of TENS (Transcutaneous Electrical Nerve Stimulation) under medication

Time	Activity	Pain amount	Pain place	Medication	Mood
10.00	Sitting	7	Lower back	2 co-proxamol	6
11.00	Made coffee	5	Lower back	Used TENS	3

They may be filled in by the nurse at regular intervals as part of the care plan. The pain is assessed with the patient as the patient's own estimate of pain is used as the basis for treatment. Pain assessment charts give the patient's recording of their pain at various times during the day and medication can be adjusted accordingly to give effective pain relief. Patients may also be given a pain chart or diary to fill in postoperatively following day surgery or discharge from the ward.

Visual analogue scales

Visual analogue scales (VAS) are used to measure pain, treatment satisfaction, sleep and mood. They are also used to monitor the effects of drugs. The advantages of a VAS are that it is sensitive to small changes, can be used to measure pain intensity and pain relief, and is easy for the patient to use. The VAS is a quick and easy method of scoring pain and can be used at frequent intervals. The disadvantages are that pain is only scored on a single dimension and the score is influenced by the most prominent feature of the pain. Some patient groups, e.g. the elderly or the visually impaired, may find it difficult to use. VAS consists of a 10 cm line that ranges from 'No pain' to 'Worst possible pain'. The patient or nurse then marks the point on the line to coincide with the reported level of pain. The distance from 'No pain' to the point marked is then measured and this gives a numerical score.

In the assessment of protracted or chronic pain, a body chart may be used (Figure 5.1). This consists of a simple outline of the front and back views of the body. The patient is asked to mark, on the body chart, the location and area of the pain. Any changes can be noted on further charts and action taken to relieve the pain noted. Other forms of VAS are the pain thermometer and the horizontal scale (Figure 5.2).

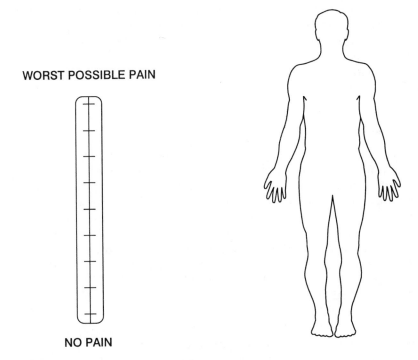

WORST POSSIBLE PAIN

NO PAIN

Figure 5.1   Example of a body chart and pain thermometer.

No pain---X-----------------------Worst possible pain

Figure 5.2   Example of a visual analogue scale.

The patient is asked to place a mark on the scale to represent the level of pain at that time. This scale can be used several times a day and a pain profile may then be constructed. This can also show the effectiveness or otherwise of treatment.

The McGill Pain Questionnaire

The McGill Pain Questionnaire (MPQ) was devised in Canada and contains sets of words that are used to quantify pain severity. There are sets of words for the categories sensory, affective, evaluative and miscellaneous. Words in each category that indicate the quality and severity of the pain are selected by the patient.

From these responses a **pain rating index** (PRI) is calculated. This is based on a numerical value ascribed to each word, 1 indicating mild pain and 5 excruciating pain. The questionnaire provides a comprehensive analysis of pain and is used in many pain clinics. However, as it is a lengthy questionnaire to administer it is not ideal for repeated use with chronic sufferers. Many therapists and clinics now use the short-form MPQ, which is easy to administer and can easily be repeated at a later date.

Performance testing

The assessments used for testing performance should be suitable for use as an objective measure of relative ability and any difficulty experienced when carrying out an activity. The assessment should provide a baseline upon which to monitor progress on reassessment – a framework within which to discuss the implications of functional difficulty with both patients and relatives. It should also provide a framework within which to plan and evaluate both physiotherapy and occupational therapy treatment programmes or interventions.

When the patient is assessed initially their performance levels are assessed by the therapist. The therapist looks at the sitting, standing and walking tolerance of the patient and their ability to carry out everyday tasks. Some of the tests used are a timed walk test and various stamina tests such as stair-climbing, sit-to-stand repetitions and step-ups. This assessment may be carried out by the physiotherapist or occupational therapist, as many pain teams have combined assessments that can be carried out by any member of the pain team.

Timed walk test

The timed walk test is carried out over a set distance. Usually the patient is asked to complete the walk as quickly as they can. If the patient normally uses a walking stick then they may be allowed to use this aid. The patient may stop for a rest but this is included in the test time. The time registered is the total time the patient takes to complete the test. This test gives an indication of the patient's current mobility level, how long they can walk without a rest and how much activity they are taking on a regular basis. Pain behaviours such as leaning against walls, holding the limb and verbalization are noted, as is the type of walking aid used. Some therapists encourage patients to carry out this test without aids.

Step test

The step test to tolerance in 1 minute is performed on a step bench; the patients are asked to perform as many step-ups in 1 minute as they can. If the patient is unable to complete the 1 minute test the limiting factor is recorded – i.e. whether it is pain or lack of cardiovascular endurance. This test is based on the functional activity of stair-climbing, as the step-up bench is approximately the same height as a normal step. This also gives an indication of the stamina level of the patient. Sometimes a 3-minute step test may be used as a baseline for fitness. If a flight of stairs is available in the clinic, then this may be incorporated into the test.

Stamina

Stamina is 'staying power', that is the length of time an exercise or activity can be maintained. Pain affects all areas of physical activity, from work activities to daily activities such as getting in and out of a chair or going up and down stairs. To improve stamina and fitness it is recommended that 20-minute sessions of aerobic exercise are carried out three times a week. This involves sustained rhythmic movement of the large muscles, using oxygen for energy. When increasing stamina by regular exercise progress can be monitored by taking the pulse rate before and after exercise. As stamina levels improve the pulse rate should return to normal more quickly.

Schmidt (1985a, b) carried out a series of studies that looked at the performance of chronic low back pain patients during standardized back stress tests. He found that the patients who only received feedback on their performance did not show any increase in pain. However the group who received feedback but also had high performance demands reported a significant increase in pain. In one study using a treadmill exercise test subjects could not see a clock and had no information or feedback on their performance. They had to make the decision to stop the exercise with no external aids and, in comparison with the control group, they consistently overestimated the amount of exercise they had taken. This illustrates the importance of feedback on performance so that the patient can learn to monitor and improve their own fitness levels.

Many pain clinics use a video to record the patients' initial and end of course activity assessment. Others may use the video to film the first and last exercise sessions of a group. The video is then shown to the patients at the end of the course, enabling them to see for themselves the difference in mobility and ease of movement between the beginning and end of the course. There is always some improvement, even if it is only in the patient's confidence to move without guarding the body against pain. This presents as a more fluid body movement as opposed to a stiff, guarded movement. Keefe and Block (1982) carried out studies which looked at pain behaviour in a standardized setting. They used a video to record behaviours while the patient engaged in activities likely to increase pain, such as sitting, standing, walking and lying. They found that this was a reliable method and that motor pain behaviours such as guarding, bracing, rubbing of the painful area, sighing and grimacing were a valid index of pain.

Questionnaires

The patient may fill in questionnaires relating to activity levels. The most commonly used are the Oswestry Low Back Disability Questionnaire (Fairbank *et al.*, 1980) and the Sickness Impact Profile (Bergner *et al.*, 1976).

The Oswestry Low Back Disability Questionnaire

The Oswestry Low Back Disability Questionnaire covers pain intensity, personal care, lifting, walking, sitting, standing, sleeping, sex life, social life and travelling. The self-administered questionnaire avoids any interviewer bias and ensures uniformity of presentation. The combination of closed questions and self-administration gives a reliable format (Collen *et al.*, 1969). The subsequent disability score is used as a guide to a patient's treatment programme. It cannot be used in isolation, since it makes no allowance for the demands of a patient's job, their age, or their psychological make-up.

Sickness impact profile

This scale was intended to measure overall severity of disability, i.e. the extent to which an individual's performance of activities is limited by impairment. The Sickness Impact Profile is very detailed and covers all aspects of daily life, working life and social life. It also incorporates questions relating to psychological well-being, for example, questions on sleep, confusion and anxiety. Some of the questions also relate to communication and eating. This questionnaire is very broad in the areas it covers and, although very thorough, filling it in can lead to questionnaire fatigue. Each section has an overall score and this has led to sections, for instance on mobility and self-care, being used in isolation. The patient only ticks the statement on the questionnaire that is applicable to them personally.

ASSESSMENT OF FUNCTION

'Function' in this context refers to the ability to carry out activities in everyday life or those activities needed for the work and social environment. Jette (1985) said that function could be divided into four categories: 'physical function, mental function, emotional function and social function'. However as the terms 'activities of daily living' (ADL) and 'functional performance' have become synonymous, Pedretti's (1985) definition of ADL as 'tasks of self maintenance, mobility, communication and home management that enable an individual to achieve personal independence in his or her environment' is a more accurate description of function. The patient can be assessed by observation of the way they walk into the pain clinic or assessment room. For example: are they leaning heavily on a walking stick or their partner's arm; are they in a wheelchair; are they wearing aids as well as using them (collar, splint, corset, etc.); are they exhibiting pain behaviours through their body language?

Basic activity assessment

This assessment is based on activities which are easy to carry out, do not require extensive equipment and are closely related to ADL. This may consist of one task or several. A six-point activity test (Figure 5.3) consists of six activities: getting on/off a chair; getting on/off a bed (patient has to lie down); picking a pen off the floor; putting on/taking off a shoe; going through a heavy swing door, so that the pain or level of independence can be measured in pushing/pulling; and a step up.

Date			
On/off chair			
On/off bed			
Take shoe off/on			
Go through swing door			
Step up			
Pick pen up from floor			

Figure 5.3 Six-point activity test. Scoring key: 1 = Independent without help or aids; 2 = Independent with some difficulty; 3 = Has difficulty and sometimes needs help; 4 = Always needs help; 5 = Unable to carry out task.

These activities are scored on a scale of 1–5, 1 being 'independent' and 5 'unable to carry out the task'. The same equipment is used for each patient and the patient is measured on their ability to carry out the task irrespective of disability, age or pain. Observations of any pain behaviours while the patient is carrying out these simple tasks can be noted.

A single activity task could be to make a cup of coffee. This would incorporate various movements such as reaching up into the cupboard to get cups out, bending down to the fridge to get the milk and carrying the kettle to the sink to fill it. This type of activity could be videoed so that the patient's task analysis, their posture and pacing of activity could be observed and recorded. Some therapists use very simple timed tasks such as putting on a pair of shoes with laces. Again, any pain behaviours are observed and recorded.

Subjective activity questionnaire

It is also useful to get the patient to fill in a simple questionnaire on pain in relation to activity. Therapists tend to use a list of everyday activities which the
patients are asked to score on a pain scale of 0–5. Although this is subjective, it
gives the therapist an indication of the patient's perception of their pain in relation to everyday activity. The questionnaire that appears to be most commonly
used (Table 5.4) is based on 14, activities which are scored on a pain scale of
0–5 where 0 is 'pain-free' and 5 'Most painful'.

Some activities are repeated but have a distraction element added, e.g.
sitting/watching TV and standing/washing up. Some information can be
collected from questionnaires such as the Oswestry Low Back Pain Disability
Questionnaire and the Sickness Impact Profile. Currently the special interest
group (Occupational Therapists in Pain Management) are evaluating and modifying the current assessments used with the aim of devising a tool which can be
used as an evaluation and outcome measure.

Table 5.4   Example of subjective activity questionnaire

Activity	Pain-free 0	Slight pain 1	Slight pain 2	Painful 3	Painful 4	Most painful 5
Sitting						
Standing						
Pick up from floor						
Hang out washing						
Washing up						
Put socks or tights on						
Cut toenails						
Ironing						
Bath/shower						
Driving						
Walking						
Lying down						
Sleeping						
Watching TV						

Summary

Assessments are used to evaluate performance and these are made by interview,
observation and written information from the patient in the form of questionnaires. The aims of assessment are to find baselines for activity in relation to
pain, to assess levels of functional independence, posture and ease of movement. This can be carried out as previously mentioned, but in addition to this a
structured interview can prove useful.

Structured interview

In some pain clinics assessment interviews are carried out jointly by the occupational therapist and the physiotherapist. This saves time and means that the patient is not taken over the same ground by several different people. The interview can establish how much help the patient is having with personal care and daily activities. It can also provide information in relation to the pain – i.e. is the pain interfering with the patient's social life and activity levels and which hobbies and activities are no longer carried out because of pain? The therapist will be able to ascertain whether the patient is still able to work or intends to return to work, the type of work and relevant working positions involved. If a patient is having difficulty performing these everyday tasks as a result of physical or mental dysfunction, the problems are identified, with the patient, by means of evaluation. Evaluation in this area consists of systematic observation and interview to determine which tasks cannot be performed and what the limiting factors are. If the limiting factors are not amenable to treatment, the therapist will show the patient alternative methods of carrying out the activity or how to compensate for these limitations.

Conclusion

The pain assessment is the starting point for treatment and enables us to see how pain is affecting the patient's lifestyle, whether there is loss of role within the family group and how the pain affects the patient in the areas of personal care and activities of daily living. It also allows the therapist to observe whether there is any pain behaviour, any abnormal gait or postures and whether any aids or equipment are used or needed.

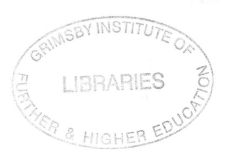

6 | Pain procedures

INTRODUCTION

Various techniques and procedures are used in the relief or treatment of chronic pain. These are usually administered by physiotherapists and doctors, although TENS, massage and cutaneous stimulation using heat or cold are also used by occupational therapists and nurses in treatment. Physical techniques such as cutaneous stimulation and massage can give pain relief, as can other methods of stimulating the skin, for example electrical stimulation. Electrotherapeutic modalities for the relief of pain cause local chemical changes in the tissues, activate the pain gate control mechanism and increase the blood flow to the area treated. Other therapeutic modalities used in the treatment of pain are nerve blocks and analgesics. Nerve blocks are used for diagnosis, prognosis and as a therapeutic treatment medium. Drugs which are used to relieve pain can alter the pain sensation, depress pain perception or modify the patient's response to pain. Generally medication is most effective if its selection is based on the cause and intensity of the pain.

PHYSICAL TECHNIQUES

In this section cutaneous stimulation, massage, manipulation, electrotherapy and hydrotherapy will be described. These techniques are used for pain relief and relaxation in the health service as well as in fitness clubs, beauty salons and alternative health clinics.

Cutaneous stimulation

Cutaneous stimulation is 'the stimulating of the skin for purposes of relieving pain' (McCaffery and Beebe, 1989). The rationale for using cutaneous stimulation is based on the gate control theory. Stimulation techniques inhibit the transmission of pain messages and increase the body's release of endorphins. During the application of cutaneous stimulation pain may be eliminated or reduced, and this effect may continue even after the stimulation has ceased. Cutaneous stimulation is used for the relief of muscle spasm, to decrease anxiety, to increase relaxation and muscle activity, to decrease pain and as a distraction technique. Techniques that are commonly used include massage, application of heat and cold, ultrasound and transcutaneous nerve stimulation (TNS). For details of different types of massage see Chapter 9 and for information on TNS see below.

Superficial temperature alteration

The application of heat or cold predominantly effects the skin and subcutaneous tissue. Sometimes the muscles can be affected but any deeper or more distal effects are indirect and due to reflex activity. Superficial heating can be achieved by using a hot water bottle, an electric heating pad, hot compresses, heat packs, a hot bath or a heat lamp. The manufacturer's instructions should be carefully followed when using any electrical equipment in the home, and hot water bottles should have a cover to prevent burns. The application of heat can reduce muscle spasm, relieve ischaemia, increase the blood flow and reduce tension in trigger points. It can also reduce joint stiffness, pain sensitivity and increase muscle relaxation.

The effects of superficial cooling last longer than heating and can be achieved using cold compresses, frozen gel packs and flexible cold packs. Cool packs should always be wrapped with a cloth and should not be placed directly on the skin. The application of cold reduces muscle spasm and can reduce or prevent bleeding through vasoconstriction. Cold also reduces sensitivity by lowering the temperature of nerve fibres and receptors.

Contrast bathing by immersing the limb alternately in hot and cold baths can also help in pain relief. This technique is inappropriate for acute trauma and bleeding, and cold applications, which reduce muscle spasm and increase vasoconstriction, are more suitable in these situations. The application of heat may increase the risk of bleeding through vasodilation. Contrast bathing is also contraindicated for patients with impaired sensation or numbness as the patient is unable to identify when the temperature level is excessive, thus risking further tissue damage.

Icing is often used as a counter-irritant, to produce numbness or anaesthesia, to deactivate trigger points and for stimulation of acupuncture points. It should be used in short bursts of 10 minutes maximum to avoid tissue damage. Icing is sometimes used by therapists prior to activity or movement of a limb.

Ultrasound

This method raises the temperature in deep structures. Pressure waves are produced at high frequencies of over 1 million Hz. When these are focused and beamed they will travel through water and soft tissue like an intense beam of light, which is absorbed. When the sound waves reach the bone they are converted to heat, producing a localized deep heat. Ultrasound is used in the treatment of joint stiffness.

Electrotherapy

Ultrasound (see above), H-wave, laser therapy, pulsed shortwave and interferential currents are used in the treatment of painful conditions.

H-wave

H-wave causes both muscular and neuromuscular stimulation. A high- or low-frequency impulse can be used either over or near the injury site. The low-frequency impulses cause muscular contractions, which increase blood flow and stimulate the lymphatic drainage of an injury site. This in turn accelerates the removal of pain-producing chemicals and toxins which have built up around the injury site, reducing pain and stimulating the body's healing processes. High-frequency impulses cause deep analgesia and stimulate the body's natural pain-reducing chemicals, which close the pain gate.

H-wave is contraindicated if the patient has a pacemaker or any other electrical implant and also in conditions such as acute phlebitis, epilepsy, pregnancy, deep vein thrombosis or undiagnosed pain. The pads should not be placed across the heart, the brain or the carotid artery. Sometimes H-wave may cause nausea or faintness. If the patient has recently taken alcohol H-wave is not recommended.

Laser therapy

Laser therapy is used in the treatment of pain by application of the laser source to trigger acupuncture points. Continuous or pulsed output at different frequencies can be used for tissue healing and pain control. A low- or medium-power laser is used and this can be hand-held or used with a stand.

Pulsed shortwave

Pulsed shortwave is used in the treatment of painful conditions such as reflex sympathetic dystrophy, phantom limb pain, causalgia and osteoporotic pain. Diapulse and megapulse are commonly used.

Interferential currents

Interferential current therapy is based on a principle of two alternating currents which are passed, slightly out of phase, through the tissues. It is said to cause the release of enkephalins and endorphins when a low frequency is used, while the high-frequency current causes temporary inhibition of fibres, which closes the pain gate. Although it is said to be effective in the treatment of pain there is little objective evidence to support this theory.

Hydrotherapy

Historically people have attended health spas which had warm water springs or mineral waters to relieve their aches and pains. Hydrotherapy is the use of warm water for therapeutic purposes. Many hospitals and clinics have hydrotherapy pools for supervised treatment sessions. There are several properties of the water that aid pain relief. These are buoyancy, hydrostatic pressure, turbulence and temperature. The buoyancy of the water aids muscle relaxation, mobility and pain relief. Hydrostatic pressure increases the flow of venous blood and lymph, which aids oedema reduction and pain relief. Water turbulence is used to ease tension and pain and the temperature of the water induces relaxation, relieves muscle spasm, increases the circulation and facilitates movement and mobility. This has a psychological as well as a physiological effect, in that the pain patient is able to move easily in the water without increasing their pain. Some clinics may have whirlpool baths, where the agitation of the water acts as cutaneous stimulation. Some pain sufferers find that Jacuzzi or spa baths can aid relaxation and pain relief.

Manipulation

This can be provided by osteopaths, chiropractors (Chapter 9) or physiotherapists. Manipulation is the use of manual pressure on the spine and soft tissues to relieve pain and discomfort. Dr James Cyriax from St Thomas' Hospital, London began to teach physiotherapy students how to use his manipulative techniques (Cyriax and Cyriax, 1984) in the 1940s. Manipulation techniques involve the application of high-velocity low-amplitude thrusts. The aim of manipulation is to restore normal mobility to joints which have restricted movement and associated dysfunction. It is also used to relieve pain and muscle spasm. Manipulation causes stimulation of the mechanoreceptors which block the pain messages to the brain and give relief.

MEDICATION

Analgesics are commonly used in the relief of both chronic and acute pain, often with other treatments or therapies. They may be administered orally, intravenously or by intramuscular injection. A wide range of drugs are used by doctors in the treatment of pain. These range from simple painkillers, available at the chemist, which may help in acute episodes, to drugs for specific conditions, such as chymopapain, used in certain cases of disc protrusion.

Drugs that are used to relieve pain work in several ways: by altering the pain sensation, depressing pain perception or modifying the patient's response to pain. As a general principle drugs are used most effectively if their selection is based on the cause and intensity of pain. If pain is constant then analgesia will need to be given at regular intervals based on the drug's duration of action. If pain is episodic analgesia should be given as soon as the pain begins rather than waiting until it is unbearable.

In acute pain analgesics are used as part of the pain control regimen, which may include the teaching of breathing techniques or a basic relaxation method. In the control of postoperative pain, for instance in hip or knee replacements, patient-controlled analgesia systems are used. These work on the principle that the individual who experiences the pain is the best judge of when they need medication. The patient is able to administer analgesics as and when they need it so that they remain comfortable and pain-free during the initial recovery period. Patients using this system of medication must be able to understand instructions, able to manage the technical aspects of a pump and confident about handling their own medication. The patient is able to stay in control of their pain and regular medication can be administered before the pain occurs or increases.

In chronic pain analgesia is used for the relief of persistent pain. In the case of malignant chronic pain, where life expectancy is short, the analgesia prescribed should be of sufficient strength, quantity and frequency to control the pain (Lipton, 1979). For patients with persistent pain and a normal life expectancy psychotropic drugs, such as antidepressants (which are effective when there is evidence of strong emotional or psychological factors affecting the pain) and tranquillizers, are sometimes used to relieve the pain. These drugs mainly affect synaptic transmission in the CNS. In chronic pain treatment drugs are most commonly used in conjunction with other coping strategies to maximize pain control and quality of life.

The drugs used in pain control can be broadly categorized into analgesics and adjuvant therapy. **Analgesics** are drugs that directly induce a state of analgesia whereas **adjuvants** may not have analgesic properties in their own right but, when used in combination with other conventional analgesics, they can significantly help with pain control or relief.

Analgesics

Analgesics act in the brain, spinal cord, nerve endings and at the site of tissue damage to reduce the amount of pain being felt. They are sometimes classified as mild, moderate and strong analgesics. Mild analgesics are usually drugs such as aspirin and paracetamol, which can be bought at the chemist or supermarket. Moderate analgesics are drugs such as codeine, dihydrocodeine and co-proxamol. Morphine and buprenorphine are usually referred to as strong analgesics. Analgesics are selective as they are able to diminish pain without affecting other sensations. They can be divided into two groups: non-opiates and opiates.

Non-steroidal anti-inflammatory drugs

Non-steroidal anti-inflammatory drugs (NSAIDs) are effective for mild to moderate pain and have three effects: analgesic, anti-inflammatory and antipyretic. They are generally considered to work at a peripheral level by inhibiting prostaglandin synthesis and preventing sensitization of pain receptors to pain. They are used as general analgesics and for conditions where pain is directly related to bony disease or damage, e.g. arthritis and bony metastases. Possible side effects of this group of drugs are gastric irritation and ulceration, bleeding and renal insufficiency, which can be a limiting factor on usage. Often drugs such as antacids or cimetidine (which reduce gastric irritation) are given concurrently with NSAIDs. NSAIDs are available in short-acting or slow-release preparations. Indomethacin and aspirin are also available in suppository form. Commonly used NSAIDs are indomethacin, ibuprofen and naproxen. To counteract the tendency of this group of drugs to cause gastric irritation and bleeding, patients are advised to take their medication with food, or an alternative drug from this group may be tried until the patient finds one that suits them.

Opiate analgesics

This group of drugs is used for the treatment of moderate to severe pain and may be used in combination with NSAIDs and/or co-analgesics. Opiates work by binding to the opiate receptors in the central nervous system. As the opiate analgesics vary in opiate receptor site binding they vary in action and side effects. Dosage is limited by the side effects. Opiate analgesics can be divided into three groups:

- opium derivatives (morphine and codeine);
- semi-synthetic derivatives (oxycodone and diamorphine);
- synthetic analgesics (pethidine and methadone).

The drugs most commonly used for severe pain are morphine, diamorphine and pethidine.

Opiate analgesics vary in their potency. The choice of opiate analgesic is based on the type of pain (acute or chronic), ease of administration (route and dosing interval), the individual patient response to the drug, known side effects and the length of anticipated use.

Drugs such as morphine and pethidine suppress the affective, autonomic and motor aspects of pain. They act centrally on the opiate receptors in the CNS. Receptors are found in the midbrain (PAGM), and the dorsal horn and forebrain. Pethidine is not recommended for prolonged episodes of acute or chronic pain because of its short duration of action (2–3 h) and the high incidence of side effects. Morphine is available in varying concentrations of short-acting tablets, sustained-release tablets and liquid preparations, which can be used for oral administration. Suppositories are also available. Diamorphine and morphine can be used in subcutaneous injections or infusions via a syringe driver and intravenous injections or continuous infusions via an intravenous infusion pump. Nausea, vomiting and constipation are common side effects.

The stronger opiate analgesics can cause some depression of the respiratory centre. Patients do, however, develop tolerance to the respiratory depression and, as long as patients undergoing opiate therapy are carefully monitored, problems can be avoided. Adequate analgesia without drowsiness is the optimal goal for pain management, although it is not always achievable. Long-term use of analgesics may lead to a decreasing response (**tolerance**) to the prescribed dose as well as to physical dependence. In this situation the individual may experience withdrawal symptoms if medication is stopped. This can be managed by altering the dosage or changing the analgesic. However a study carried out in the Yom Kippur War (Melzack and Wall, 1991) found that when narcotics were given for pain relief there was no indication of addiction; similarly cancer patients who take regular doses for months or years show no sign of tolerance to these drugs.

Problems with analgesics

One possible problems with analgesics as medication is that the effect may only last for 2–3 h and if the patient waits until the first dose has worn off before taking the next tablet they may need a bigger dose to get on top of the pain again. Secondly, every time the effect of the drug wears off, the falling blood concentration can give withdrawal sensations. Thirdly, the body may learn to expect pain every 2–3 h. Finally, if analgesics are taken every 2–3 h for long periods it may result in damage to the liver or kidneys.

Possible solutions

The use of long-acting drugs, such as codeine, dihydrocodeine and co-proxamol, can overcome the short-term effect of analgesics, as these last for 8–12 h. Analgesics can be used as a preventative measure by taking the medication before the pain builds up and the pain cycle starts. They can also be used in conjunction with other methods of pain relief, enabling gradual reduction of analgesics as the patient becomes proficient in these other coping techniques or strategies.

Other drugs used to relieve pain

Other drugs used in pain relief are antidepressants, anticonvulsants, sedatives and tranquillizers.

Antidepressants

This group of drugs has been found to be effective in treatment of specific types of pain when used in low doses. They work by altering the balance of pain-transmitting substances in the brain and spinal cord. Drugs most commonly prescribed are amitriptyline and clomipramine.

The side effects are drowsiness, a dry mouth and occasionally blurred vision or difficulty in passing urine. These drugs are best taken at night, as this minimizes the side effects.

Anticonvulsants

Some pains caused by nerve damage can be helped by anticonvulsants at a low dosage. Anticonvulsants work by reducing the sensitivity of the damaged nerves. Drugs most commonly prescribed are carbamazepine and sodium valproate. Some people react badly to this group of drugs. They feel very ill and can also have gastric problems and skin rashes. This is generally avoided by starting the patient on a very low dosage and gradually increasing the amount taken.

Sedatives, tranquillizers and sleeping tablets

This group of drugs should only be used for short periods for relieving stress. The one most commonly prescribed is diazepam. This group of drugs is very addictive. If the patient stops them suddenly they will tend to feel more anxious and have difficulty sleeping. They should be reduced gradually under medical supervision. To avoid addiction the medication should be taken for as short a time as possible. The patient should be counselled about the possibility of side effects and given support when reducing the dosage. They should be encouraged to use other methods of relieving stress such as relaxation and physical activity.

Adjuvant therapy

The most commonly used adjuvant therapies for pain relief include antidepressants, tranquillizers, anticonvulsants, muscle relaxants and steroids. It is only under a certain set of specific circumstances that the use of any one of these drugs is indicated.

Antidepressants can be very effective when depression and anxiety are increasing the patient's perception of pain. Similarly, lack of sleep can influence the pain perception and a mild night sedative can be effective. When muscle spasm is the cause of the pain a muscle relaxant may be prescribed. Corticosteroids are used to relieve pain caused by raised intracranial pressure and nerve compression. Anticonvulsants, antihistamines and antibiotics may be used in specific types of pain. The drugs used in adjuvant therapy for pain relief are also called 'co-analgesics'.

NERVE BLOCKS AND INJECTIONS

Injections are an accurate and effective way of delivering treatment to the source of the problem. Sometimes this form of treatment does not give immediate relief and it may take several sessions before the pain begins to diminish. The success of the treatment also depends on the patient following the doctor's advice, between treatment sessions and after the course of treatment has finished. The pain is usually unilateral and restricted to a specific area.

Muscular injections

Pain from spinal structures can radiate to surrounding areas and set up secondary points of tension, which become taut bands or knots in the muscle. These are referred to as fibrositis but are more commonly known as **trigger points** and are also called myofascial dysfunction. They commonly occur in the neck and shoulders and may be due to postural stress or an acute episode of neck pain. They may also present as postoperative or post-traumatic neuroma formations. When touched, a hard nodule is felt and when pressure is applied to the area pain is felt or increased. Trigger points are often successfully treated with a course of local injections containing a corticosteroid combined with a local anaesthetic.

Facet joint injections

Injections can be performed for localized painful joints such as a facet, shoulder, elbow, or knee joint. The same procedure is used as for localized painful trigger areas. A mixture of bupivacaine and prednisolone or methylprednisolone is commonly injected to numb the area and reduce any localized inflammation. Should longer-term therapy be required, cryotherapy, i.e. freezing of a particular area or nerve, may be useful. This procedure is usually performed on an outpatient basis under X-ray control.

Epidural injections

Epidurals offer effective pain relief for back pain or referred nerve root pain. Back pain or referred nerve root pain is commonly due to benign conditions such as osteoarthritis or osteoporosis. However, malignant disease such as spinal secondaries may also cause such symptoms and opiate therapy is administered via the epidural route for these conditions. Epidurals are also used for postoperative pain relief and labour pain. Injections into the epidural space can help in the relief of symptoms associated with disc protrusions that have not responded to bed rest, pain killers and manipulation or other physiotherapy techniques.

The injection is administered between the outer lining of the dura and the bony walls of the spinal canal. It differs from epidural given to relieve pain in childbirth in two ways. In childbirth the epidural is administered via the lower back whereas for orthopaedic cases the base of the sacrum is injected and a weaker solution of local anaesthetic and added steroid is used. The anaesthetic numbs the lining of the spinal cord, which is under pressure. The steroid helps to reduce inflammation and bruising of the dural sheath which has been caused by pressure and friction. During the injection pain can be aggravated but once the injection has finished the pain should cease. The pain relief varies from total relief to a few hours. Second or third epidurals may be given at weekly intervals if the first one only gives partial relief.

Between 40% and 70% of patients obtain some relief from epidural injections and complications are rare. A common phenomenon is that of temporary numbness and paralysis of the lower legs, this clears after a few hours. Epidurals are given under local anaesthetic, often on a day-surgery basis.

Nerve blocks

These can be an effective treatment when the cause of pain is found to be nerve irritation. An injection of local anaesthetic and steroid to the nerve root will anaesthetize the nerve and reduce any inflammation. This procedure is usually carried out by orthopaedic or pain consultants on an outpatient basis. The only risk from this injection is that occasionally the dural membrane may be pierced. If this happens the patient has to lie flat for 24 hours, as headache or dizziness caused by leak of the cerebrospinal fluid may occur. This should resolve within 2 days. Because of this minor risk patients are always advised to arrange for someone to drive them home after this procedure. If the nerve root has been successfully located the anaesthetic will provide several days' pain relief. The results are variable and it is difficult for doctors to predict how well a particular individual will respond. This procedure is sometimes used as a diagnostic tool with back problems to elicit the origin of referred pain.

Sacral intrathecal blocks

These are used for perineal pain due to rectal or pelvic tumour. Due to the close proximity of the posterior sensory and anterior motor nerves at the sacral level there can be complications. This can result in loss or impairment of bladder or bowel control.

Coeliac plexus block

This type of procedure is used in the treatment of symptoms such as pain, nausea and vomiting associated with carcinoma of the upper abdomen or diseases of the stomach, liver, pancreas and gall bladder. It is carried out under X-ray control.

Thoracic somatic paravertebral block

This procedure is used in conditions where lung or bronchial tumours are causing pressure on the chest wall and thoracic nerves, where malignant or benign bone disease causes nerve irritation and invasion, and in patients with thoracotomy scar pain. The procedure is performed under X-ray control so that the appropriate level and space can be identified with contrast medium. For diagnostic purposes a local anaesthetic such as bupivacaine is injected. For a more permanent block a neurolytic agent such as phenol glycerine is injected. This procedure can be carried out unilaterally or bilaterally. Complications are rare, but a pneumothorax is possible, because of the proximity of the injection to the lung. Blood pressures can occasionally fall, particularly with local anaesthetic.

Lumbar psoas block

This procedure is used for a painful hip or knee. It can be performed as a regional block during an operation or as a therapeutic technique for conditions such as osteoporosis, osteoarthritis, Paget's disease or bone metastases. It is usually performed at the L3 level under X-ray control, either unilaterally or bilaterally. The procedure can cause a drop in blood pressure due to accidental intravascular injection or a toxic reaction. Transient numbness and/or weakness of the lower limbs may also occur because of the involvement of sensory and motor nerve fibres. These effects are usually only temporary. The length of time during which relief is felt following this procedure is not predictable.

Stellate ganglion block

This procedure is used for conditions such as post-herpetic neuralgia, acute post-traumatic neuralgia, and tumours causing pain in the head, neck and arm. The latter usually involves the nerve distribution from the middle and inferior ganglion. Treatment is not successful once these conditions become chronic. The blocks are usually performed on an outpatient basis. A local anaesthetic such as bupivacaine is used. Neurolytic agents are not advised because of the close proximity of vital anatomy. The block is performed on the affected side. The patient is carefully monitored following the procedure for signs of Horner's syndrome, i.e. transient arm weakness, a hoarse voice and nasal congestion, which would indicate a successful cervical sympathetic ganglion block.

Brachial plexus block

This procedure is used when there is pain in the arm due to disease infiltration of the brachial plexus, for example in secondary carcinoma and injury to the brachial plexus. It is performed on an outpatient basis and is carried out through either the axillary, interscalene or supraclavicular route. Bupivacaine is usually used as this only affects the sensory nerves and at most only transient motor weakness is likely. Phenol can be used but this will affect motor function. A pneumothorax can be a complication of this procedure.

Intravenous regional blockade

The commonest indications for this procedure are sympathetic dystrophy syndrome, causalgia and Raynaud's syndrome. An intravenous cannula is introduced into the affected limb, which is then isolated using a modified Bier's block technique. Intravenous injections are made up in varying combinations and doses depending on the individual patient and the site to be treated. Drugs used include guanethidine (a sympathetic blocker) and lignocaine (a local anaesthetic). This procedure is usually performed on an outpatient basis and is used in conjunction with physiotherapy manipulation of the limb for maximum effect. There is transient loss of feeling in the limb. Colour changes may occur during treatment. These may present as mottled, colourless, blue and bright red skin, turning to pink as the blood returns to the limb when the cuff is released.

NEUROSURGERY

Surgical procedures were historically used in the treatment of chronic pain in conditions where medication could not control or help the pain or where the side effects caused the patient to become confused or drowsy. These procedures cause destruction of the neural pathways electrically, chemically or by cutting. Temporary lesions may be carried out by using a local anaesthetic or freezing the nerve. Sites which have been lesioned in chronic pain disorders are peripheral nerves, dorsal root, spinothalamic tract, thalamus and parts of the forebrain.

Peripheral nerves

The commonest procedure was the destruction of selected peripheral nerves in the CNS (Melzack and Wall, 1991). This was based on the specificity theory (Chapter 2), where it was assumed that surgical interruption of the pathways would prevent pain impulses from reaching the pain centre. It has now been shown that, although surgical procedures may appear to give pain relief postoperatively, the pain will usually recur and is often worse than it was before. Procedures currently used involve an injection of local anaesthetic to test the potential effectiveness of the proposed lesion, and then injection of a toxic substance to destroy the nerve fibres. Another procedure uses a high-frequency current which is passed through the tip of the needle which effectively burns the nerve. Prolonged blocking of the nerves can also be achieved by freezing. All these procedures can be used when the painful area is small and supplied by a single nerve.

Dorsal roots

When a large area is affected by pain or the area is close to the spine a **rhizotomy** may be used. This involves sectioning the dorsal roots, which only affects sensation, leaving the ventral roots so that movement is not lost. This is a major surgical procedure. Surgical lesions of nerve roots and ganglia result in total anaesthesia. Some patients may develop new sensations which are worse than the original pain. This is due to the generation of abnormal nerve impulses and the changes in the CNS caused by the cutting of peripheral nerves. Surgery is often used in the treatment of trigeminal neuralgia but the pain often recurs. In cancer patients spinal roots may be lesioned surgically or by chemical destruction. This procedure may be used in cancer of the thorax, abdomen or pelvis.

As the nerves contain both sensory and motor fibres the result is paralysis with muscle wasting and numbness. Variations on this that avoid the paralysis are selective lesioning of motor fibres or electrolytic heat lesions, which destroy the cells in the dorsal part of the dorsal horn. The latter procedure has been found to give pain relief in 60% patients with pain following brachial plexus avulsion and 50% of paraplegic patients with pain (Nashold, Higgins and Blumenkopf, 1985). Procedures involving chemical infiltration around the nerve root are also used. Over time the area of denervation may become hypersensitive and the patient feels a 'pins and needles' sensation which gradually increases in intensity until it becomes continuous pain. Surgical destruction of the sympathetic system has been shown to be effective in pain control. Because of the difficulty of surgery on the sympathetic ganglia, an injection of toxic substances to destroy the ganglia is usually carried out.

Cordotomy

Cordotomy, the cutting of axons in the ventrolateral spinal cord, used to be a common neurosurgical procedure for severe chronic pain. Although initially the patient has good pain relief the effect wears off over time. Although it may still be used in the terminal stages of cancer to give pain relief, cordotomy is not usually advocated for other patients. The other disadvantage of this surgical intervention is that the patient may become incontinent of urine and faeces.

Other operations

Cerebral operations for pain relief have not been very successful. Little success has been achieved using cortical lesions and, although some initial analgesia and relief has been achieved using thalamotomy, the pain returns in nearly all patients.

Research and increased knowledge of pain mechanisms has shown that surgical section of peripheral nerves has several effects. These are disruption of normal input patterns, scars and neuromas that may cause abnormal inputs and the destruction of channels that would normally be used for modifying pain input. Cordotomy has similar effects. Neurosurgeons are now using techniques that electrically stimulate nerves, spinal cord and areas of the brain rather than destroying them.

Electrical stimulation

Electrical stimulation is based on the premise that stimulation of large fibres should close the pain gate by inhibition of the small fibres. TENS (see below), dorsal column stimulation and brain stimulation are techniques commonly used. Percutaneous dorsal column stimulation is achieved by electrodes inserted on top of the dura just above the dorsal columns. The electrodes can be left *in situ* for several weeks, so that the level of pain relief can be measured over a period of time. If it is successful an operation is carried out in which the wires are attached to a radio stimulator. In a study by Urban and Nashold (1978) seven patients who had relief with a temporary implant were given a permanent implant and in the 2-year follow up only one patient had a recurrence of pain. It is thought that dorsal column stimulation re-establishes the normal balance between excitation and inhibition.

Brain stimulation has had mixed results. Hosobuchi, Adams and Linchitz (1977) carried out a study with six patients who underwent periaqueductal stimulation. Five patients with cancer reported complete pain relief and the sixth, who had facial pain, had partial relief. However, pain due to pinprick or intense radiant heat was unaffected and some studies have shown that patients can develop tolerance to continual stimulation. Good relief of chronic pain has also been found when the posterior thalamus is stimulated. These procedures are still being modified and it has been found that tolerance to stimulation can be overcome by reducing the stimulation time.

TRANSCUTANEOUS ELECTRICAL NERVE STIMULATION

Transcutaneous electrical nerve stimulation (TENS) is used for the relief of acute and chronic pain. TENS activates the nerve endings in a similar way to the application of heat or cold. It is suggested that TENS acts by stimulating the large-diameter nerve fibres and thereby closing the pain gate (Nathan and Wall, 1974). Others feel that TENS acts by blocking the primary afferent nerve fibres or by stimulating the production of endorphins, the body's natural painkillers.

There are many different types of TENS. The small models, designed for patient use, have a clip for belt attachment or they can be put in a pocket. Some electrodes are self-adhesive while others need an application of conductive gel. The unit is worn for as long as the patient can tolerate it. There are also special pads and tape that can be used for patients with sensitive skin.

The TENS system consists of a battery-powered electronic pulse generator. This has two or four leads connected to it, which end in electrodes that are placed on the skin. Although there are recommended placement sites, for many patients it is a question of trial and error. Many manufacturers recommend that the electrodes should be placed directly on the pain site, but if this does not bring adequate relief the electrodes should be moved to the next largest nerve that has distribution into the painful area. The stimulation is felt by the patient as a tingling or buzzing sensation. This is adjusted by the knobs on the side of the unit. The equipment should not allow prolonged muscle reaction such as twitching or spasm with stimulation.

With chronic pain the results are variable with TENS. Some patients find relief while others have none. TENS is also used for the relief of postoperative pain and there are special TENS units for use during childbirth. In the latter cases the patient should be made familiar with the units prior to operation or delivery. TENS can be used in conjunction with other therapies, such as mobilization of a joint. In acute pain this combined approach may give the best results. Treatment should be on a daily or alternate day basis for about 20–60 min per session. Sometimes prolonged or continuous treatment may be required. If there is a reaction to the treatment then it should be applied for shorter periods and less frequently.

Contraindications

The use of TENS is contraindicated if the patient has a pacemaker. Currents should not be passed over the chest or the throat, in order not to induce laryngeal spasm, neither should currents be passed through the eye. A current should not be passed through the carotid bodies or over traumatized or anaesthetic skin. TENS should not be used in pregnancy, but this does not apply to the special models intended for use during labour.

Indication for the use of TENS

Chronic pain conditions such as osteoarthritis, root pain and low back pain of unknown aetiology are common indicators for the use of TENS. It is also effective in the treatment of acute pain (including sports injuries), all types of acute sprains and joint pains. TENS can also be used in the treatment of headaches, including migraine, and neuralgias, including trigeminal, post-herpetic and atypical neuralgias. Phantom limb pain and postoperative pain can also be helped by TENS. TENS can be used in chest physiotherapy to produce bronchodilation. TENS also aids muscle relaxation and is often used prior to manipulative procedures and treatment by therapists.

Coping strategies

The individual's inability to cope with stress can affect their potential energy levels, performance, interpersonal relationships and health problems. Lazarus and Folkman (1984) stated that coping is 'a constantly changing cognitive and behavioural effort to manage specific external and/or internal demands that are appraised as taxing or exceeding the resources of the person'. This chapter also includes some practical activities for the reader to use with patients.

STRESS MANAGEMENT

The stress and tension that many people have in their lives can be reduced in two ways. The first way is to avoid, eliminate or modify the stimuli responsible for the problem. Stress can be eliminated or modified by avoiding the situations that cause it. Other environmental changes may not remove the stress, but may make it easier to cope with. This approach has limitations, as all the factors associated with the stress and strain of modern living cannot be removed. Minor adjustments to the home environment can aid relaxation but there is little that can be done to reduce the major stress-producing features in society at large. If the environment cannot be changed the individual has to learn to cope more effectively. The individual's reaction to external and internal stimuli has to be altered or modified.

The immediate environment can be altered by reducing clutter, bringing more order to the home or work. For some people it might involve a change of job, moving to a different neighbourhood, or taking up some form of regular exercise or hobby class. Avoidance of too many important life changes in a 12-month period may help, as will pacing of activities and reducing workloads. Many life events are outside the individual's control and in this case it is possible to minimize the cumulative effects of them by paying attention to general health, diet and maintaining adequate levels of exercise and sleep.

It is possible to modify reactions to stimuli when the causes of stress, the stress stimuli, cannot be altered. Relaxation is nature's antidote to stress and is one way of modifying the stress reaction.

RELAXATION

The relaxation response is the opposite of the stress response. In the same way that the stress response can become a habit, relaxation can be also become a habit. Relaxation is useful in many ways: it can lower stress levels and break the vicious circle between pain and stress. With practice the physical sensations that accompany the stress response, can be controlled, breaking the spiralling sensation of tension and stress which feed into and enhance the pain response.

Relaxation techniques enable the individual to cope with the symptoms of the stress response in particular situations. Once the individual is able to recognize the symptoms of stress and tension they will be able to control them using breathing techniques and the relaxation response. These techniques assist in the control of situations that would normally escalate the stress response or increase pain levels. The individual, not the pain, has the control. Relaxation enables the individual to function more efficiently. Relaxed people are better communicators and are usually more efficient.

Philips (1988) carried out a study of pain clinic patients which looked at the effects of relaxation training. The results showed a significant reduction in sensory and affective pain dimensions and pain intensity. A study carried out in chronic low back pain patients (Strong, 1991) used the McGill Pain Questionnaire (MPQ) to monitor progress during relaxation training. The MPQ was administered on admission, at discharge and at follow-up. The discharge results showed a decrease in all aspects of pain measured by the MPQ. However, at follow-up the pain scores were significantly increased in all areas except present pain intensity and the sensory pain index rating. Although the results were similar to the Philips study at discharge, the follow-up results indicated that the effects of relaxation training were not maintained. Strong suggests that this could be due to extraneous factors such as medication and other treatments. A number of studies have evaluated the effectiveness of relaxation (Keable, 1985; Clarke, Allard and Baybrooks, 1987) and have found that relaxation techniques can help rheumatoid arthritis sufferers more than drugs and physiotherapy. Jackson (1991) states that the individual is made aware of their body posture and is able to regain control over their body and conserve energy through relaxation. The best results are obtained when relaxation is taught in combination with exercise techniques and education in relation to pain and adaptation of the environment. Relaxation can be successful as a single therapy with back pain if the pain is not too intense.

How do we achieve relaxation?

This section will look at some techniques which can be used to achieve the relaxation response. They include **diaphragmatic breathing, deep muscle relaxation, self-hypnosis** and **autogenic techniques**.

Basic guidelines

The above techniques are four different ways of achieving the same response. If relaxation is used regularly the stress response can be kept under control. Diaphragmatic breathing is most effective if used regularly throughout the day in achieving stress control.

Relaxation should be practised at least once every day and each technique should be practised for approximately 3–4 weeks before moving on to the next technique. A regular time for relaxation practice should be set aside, and the room should be quiet and warm. Clothes should be comfortable and any tight clothing should be loosened before starting the relaxation. Relaxation should be carried out on a fairly empty stomach, **not** just after a meal.

Many people find that relaxation initially makes them sleepy; this improves with practice and eventually the patient should be able to relax and feel fresh and alert at the end of a session. It is not a good idea to carry out the relaxation last thing at night as the patient will fall asleep and not benefit from the learning process.

Diaphragmatic breathing

One of the effects of the stress response is to increase the breathing rate. When the body is stressed it works harder and needs more oxygen. This increases the breathing rate, which becomes fast and shallow. This fast or 'overbreathing' happens frequently in people who are susceptible to stress. Diaphragmatic breathing is a form of deep breathing and because it is so simple it can be carried out at any time and in any place.

Diaphragmatic breathing involves the use of the diaphragm. When a long, slow, deep breath is taken in, the lungs are filled with air and the diaphragm pulls down to allow them to expand fully. This results in the stomach swelling out as the breath is taken in and flattening again as the breath is released out. If there is no movement in the stomach this means that all the breathing is happening in the upper part of the chest which increases the tension levels as the breathing is only shallow. This technique, used regularly, can prevent the build up of stress and tension in the body. It can also be used to reduce stress levels. One or two breaths every half an hour throughout the day is recommended. It is best to link this in to the daily routine as it is then easier to remember to practise the technique. Initially, people may find it difficult to remember to practise the breaths every half an hour: various memory aids can be used such as a loose elastic band on the wrist, wearing a watch or ring on the opposite side to which they are normally worn or coloured stickers around the house.

ACTIVITY: DIAPHRAGMATIC BREATHING

Make yourself comfortable in a sitting or lying position. Place your hands on your stomach and take a deep breath. You should feel your stomach expand and your hands move outwards. Now slowly breathe out. When you breathe in imagine the air is filling up a balloon and when you breathe out the balloon is deflating.

Deep muscle relaxation

The ability to relax your skeletal muscles gives a practical point of control over the stress response. Muscle tension is a sign of an aroused state of the organism, but when tension in the muscles is low, arousal everywhere else is low. Muscle relaxation and a calm state of body and mind go hand in hand. Muscle relaxation is a neuromuscular skill which is learned through daily practice. Learning is achieved by developing our kinaesthetic sense, i.e. the sense by which we are aware of tension or relaxation in the muscles.

Muscle contraction is part of normal everyday activity; without it our muscles would soon atrophy and become useless. By learning to recognize tension in the body muscles and the face, and the sensation of relaxation in the muscles we can have more control over the stress response. Edmund Jacobson (1962) pioneered research into the relationship between muscle tension and anxiety. He realized that by relaxing the skeletal muscles both body and mind would become calmer and the tension responsible for causing illness and impeding recovery would be reduced. He developed the system of progressive relaxation, in which muscles are tensed and relaxed, group by group, throughout the body.

Many people feel that they are relaxed already, but it may be that they are used to working with high levels of tension in their muscles and have forgotten what it feels like to totally relax their muscles. Learning to recognize tension and to relax is a skill and it needs to be practised at least once a day for several weeks. If tensing any group of muscles causes pain it means that there is already an increased level of tension in that group of muscles and in this situation the individual should concentrate on relaxing that group of muscles and not tensing them. (For an example of a deep muscle relaxation script see Appendix 7A.) Relaxation, like sleep, is attained through an indirect approach.

Self-hypnosis techniques

Thinking is the most important part of the stress response. Like the physical part of the stress response, types of thinking that trigger the stress response can become a habit. These habits can be counteracted by learning to recognize them. Self-hypnosis techniques are used to relax the mind, which can help to decrease the experience of pain or other symptoms. This technique is a form of relaxation using imagery. When the body is physically relaxed, thinking about experiences or places that are associated with being relaxed and happy (e.g. a beach in the sun, being by the sea, in the countryside or in a beautiful garden) can help to relax the mind.

The chief value of hypnotherapy is that the patient relaxes deeply and passively takes in and tends to actualize the suggestions of the hypnotist, or in self-hypnosis one's own instructions. The limitations are that some people do not appear to be hypnotizable even in self-hypnosis. Present-day methods of training in this technique are based on the verbal suggestion of deep relaxation and sleep (Benson, 1976; Hewitt, 1985).

ACTIVITY: RELAXATION IMAGERY

Using your imagination, close your eyes and imagine a favourite place: a sunny beach or being in a garden full of flowers.

Whatever you choose to think about, use all your senses. Look around at the colours, experience the feelings on your face and body, the sounds and smells. When you are focusing on feelings of warmth, you could imagine a comfortable warm place (for example lying in front of an open fire) or warm colours such as red and orange.

ACTIVITY: COUNTING BACKWARDS

Close your eyes and relax. Now count slowly down from 300 to 1. This may help to relax you; it also helps with concentration. At the same time, you might imagine yourself on a slow escalator gently taking you into deeper relaxation with each breath you take.

ACTIVITY: DISTRACTING THOUGHTS

If you are troubled with distracting thoughts you might imagine your worries and problems as bubbles in a glass of carbonated water. Let yourself relax as you see the bubbles gently rise to the surface and burst, releasing all your problems and worries into the air.

ACTIVITY: SELF-HYPNOSIS TECHNIQUES

Imagine scenes that you find good to think about and easy to picture in your mind. Think of two scenes, a relaxation scene and a competency scene. For example:

- *Relaxation scene: Imagine yourself lying on a hot beach, going for a walk in the country.*

- *Competency scene: Imagine yourself doing something you are good at, such as cooking, driving, a sport, looking after children, craftwork, etc.*

Now relax yourself as far as you can, then practise imagining your scenes for a while. Experience all the details as if you were there. The next stage is to use the scenes to turn off worrying or stress-induced thoughts, or thoughts about your pain. Think about a situation that makes you feel only a little stressed, as this will be easier to control. Imagine a sequence of scenes, practising switching from the stressed thoughts to your relaxation or competency scene. Each scene should last roughly 30 seconds. When you have mastered this stress scene go on to try one that makes you feel a little more stressed. With practice you can learn to use a worrying or stress-inducing thought as a signal to 'Think relaxed', just as you can use an awareness of being physically stressed as a signal to relax physically.

Autogenic relaxation

This technique has been used since the 1920s by many physicians and psychiatrists. This technique was used by Dr Johannes H. Schultz (Schultz and Luthe, 1969) who called it 'autogene training', which means 'self-originated'. It was intended as a self-help technique following initial instruction by the doctor or therapist. Awareness is directed to the part of the body most in need of healing influence and this is given pictorial expression in the mind and reinforced by positive self-talk. Some psychiatrists use autogenics to relax the patient deeply and to help release buried memories and feelings.

Parts of the autogenic training resemble yoga or biofeedback. It involves concentration on certain physiological functions that are normally regulated only by the autonomic or involuntary nervous system. Examples of self-suggestions given are 'My right hand is becoming warmer' or 'My heartbeat is calm and strong'. Rises in hand temperature up to 10°F (1.8°C) have been recorded in trainees (Hewitt, 1985).

This technique uses the mind rather than the body, but shows the interaction between mind and body, or physical and psychological processes. When the body is tense the muscles are working and so they require more oxygen and create more waste; therefore they need a better blood supply. However, the blood is directed away from the extremities to the major muscle groups when the body is tense. This results in cold hands and feet. This reduced peripheral circulation is there all the time as a result of raised tension levels and stress.

For relaxation to occur muscle tension must be reduced and peripheral circulation increased. Experiments carried out in the 1960s with biofeedback machines found that anyone can learn to influence body systems that are normally controlled automatically. Heartbeat can therefore be controlled through conscious thought. Biofeedback is a means of monitoring body functions and systems. In the same way that the circulation can be influenced by concentrating on it, by concentrating on the hand feeling warmer you can also affect body temperature. Autogenic relaxation involves the use of feelings of warmth and heaviness in different parts of the body. It takes practice, but many people have found that it provides a useful means of relaxing and maintaining relaxation.

The benefit of this technique is that it can be used to improve the circulation in areas where healing is required or pain needs to be relieved. In autogenic training, awareness is passive and poised as it is in meditation. With practice, concentration on particular parts of the body can make them feel warmer or cooler.

Autogenics focuses on two aspects of the relaxation response: increased blood flow and decreased muscular tension. It does this by concentrating on two things that are experienced when relaxing: warmth; which is experienced when there is increased blood flow to the extremities such as the arms, legs, hands and feet and heaviness; which is felt when the muscles are relaxed. (For an example of an autogenic relaxation script see Appendix 7B.)

Positions for relaxation

It is important to relax in a position in which as little tension is felt as possible. For most people the most comfortable are lying or sitting postures. The neck and knees may need to be supported for greater comfort. Lying on the back with the palms of the hands facing down, elbows out and fingers separated is a comfortable position for many people. Alternatively any comfortable, supportive chair can be used for muscle relaxation if the patient prefers not to lie down.

The sitting position recommended for autogenic relaxation is as follows.

Sit with the hips and thighs towards the front of a straight-backed chair, with the feet square on the floor and the arms hanging loose. The individual should sit up straight, as if being pulled upwards from the top of the head, then relax all the muscles allowing the body to crumple straight down with the neck bent slightly forward. The hands should be placed on the legs just above the knees. The position of the hands should be adjusted until the individual is perfectly balanced, neither pulled backwards or forwards, fingers apart and relaxed.

GOAL SETTING

Pain affects the activities, thoughts and feelings of the pain sufferer (Chapter 3). The concept of pain management is that by working on change in activities, thoughts and feelings the pain can be reduced or maintained at a level which does not interfere with or control the life of the individual. Many pain sufferers have a pattern of activity which is called activity cycling. A consequence of activity cycling is that periods of activity become shorter and periods of rest longer. Goal setting and pacing are techniques which can be used to break this cycle of overactivity/underactivity.

Activity cycling

For most people with long term or chronic pain a clear pattern of activity can be recognized, this pattern is called activity cycling. Pain is the guiding factor and people tend to carry out an activity until the pain stops them. This is usually then followed by a period of rest, painkillers and feelings of depression and frustration. This cycle repeats itself time and time again. Each time it happens it reinforces the avoidance method of coping leading to reduced activity levels and increasing stiffness and weakness. Periods of activity become shorter and periods of rest longer, perpetuating the cycle.

Goal setting

A goal is an activity or aim that the individual would like to carry out or achieve. For example the goal might be to swim three lengths of the swimming pool. To achieve this goal they would need to work towards the goal in a planned and systematic way on a regular basis. The important thing to remember is that goal setting in the context of pain management is not dependent on the amount of pain the individual has. The target or goal should be set at a low level initially, i.e. at a level that is achievable on a good or bad day. This should gradually be increased as tolerance and practice improve the level of function required for the activity.

Having set the overall goal – swimming three lengths of the swimming pool – this should then be split up into mini-goals or stages. For example, if the individual is able to swim half a length without a break, an intermediate goal of one length could be set, then one and a half and so on until their long-term goal is reached. The next stage is only embarked on when the previous stage becomes easy to achieve whatever the level of pain. In this way fitness, stamina and confidence will improve over a period of time. The aim is to work in small achievable steps towards the long-term goal. People often make the steps or mini-goals too large or ambitious and then they are unable to achieve the task they have set themselves. If this happens the steps need to be broken down into smaller more manageable ones. This process may take weeks or months.

Summary

- Set goals, long-term and then short-term ones, working towards the ultimate goal.
- Establish activity baselines, i.e. how much the person is able to do without aggravating the pain.
- Adjust the goal-setting process to the person's rate of progress.
- Reinforcers or rewards help increase the frequency of a task. For most people the feeling of achievement is a reward in itself.
- Social reinforcement when it is planned with another person (e.g. friends or family) is helpful.

- Modelling: the presence of another individual doing a similar activity successfully can act as a successful model. This is one of the benefits of group participation in pain management rather than individual therapy.
- If a person's pain is increased through the activity then the goal or level of activity may need to be reassessed and worked on at a lower level.
- Pain can be minimized by setting a low baseline and not increasing too quickly. Education and reassurance about not creating damage will help to allay the person's anxieties, which in itself can have a positive effect.

PACING

When people suffer from pain for any length of time activity levels become reduced. Pain controls activity level. When teaching patients to pace their activities three things need to be considered: prioritizing, planning and pacing.

Prioritizing

The following questions need to be asked by the individual:

- Does it all need to be done today?
- Can I get someone to help me?
- Does it need to be done at all?

Having asked these questions, they may decide that the job does not need to be carried out either by themselves or at all. However, if the job does need to be carried out then the next stage is to **plan** the activity.

Planning

This involves breaking the job down into stages and looking at the things needed to carry out the job. It is better to carry out activities on the basis of 'a little and often', with regular changes of position and limited rest or relaxation periods in between. The individual should ask themselves the following questions:

- Can I break the job down into different stages?
- What do I need to carry out the job?
- What basic activities does each stage involve – e.g. walking, sitting, standing?

Many jobs can be broken down into stages, for example preparing and cooking a meal. The basic stages would be collection of ingredients (this might include going to the shops, which in turn would include walking, travelling on a bus or in a car, carrying and lifting of the shopping and possibly reaching or bending to pick up or get shopping off shelves), preparation of vegetables, etc., cooking, laying the table, serving out the meal, washing up and clearing away after the meal.

ACTIVITY

In the example above the first stage has been broken down into even smaller stages. Ask the patient to carry out a similar exercise with the other stages involved in cooking a meal.

The list of activities involved in each stage is varied and some of the activities such as walking and standing may have to be worked on as mini goals if the person's walking or standing tolerance is limited.

Pacing

How are activities paced? First a **baseline** needs to be found for each activity which causes difficulty. A baseline is the level at which an activity can be performed regularly, on good or bad days. This level can then be increased gradually (through the goal-setting process) as stamina and exercise tolerance improve.

Finding the baseline for an activity

First choose an activity – e.g. sitting. Time how long the individual is able to sit comfortably at different times during the day, take the average of these times and halve it, this is the individual's baseline for sitting. The same method can be used for walking, standing or carrying out a task.

ACTIVITY

Now choose an activity or task that you carry out frequently and work out your baseline for that activity. That baseline is the level at which you should be able to carry out your chosen activity every day regardless of any other circumstances.

A little and often is a good starting point; never try to carry out everything at once. Other aspects that can help with pacing are checking that work areas are organized in the most efficient and ergonomic way, using the correct equipment (modified if necessary – e.g. long-handled tools) so that minimum effort is expended. Goals should be practised on a regular basis and should not be set too high.

Once the tasks have been prioritized and planned the next step is to ensure that the vicious circle of overactivity and underactivity does not recur. Pacing of activities can prevent this. Tolerance levels for activity should be built up gradually and systematically. Regular rests should be taken between activities. Many people fall into the trap of pushing themselves that little bit further because then the job will be finished, the 'five minutes more' syndrome. This usually results in increased pain levels and a reduction in activity for the next few days. Positions should be changed regularly and activities planned so that rests and changes of position are included. The following example shows how a simple activity can be planned and paced using the baselines for basic activities such as standing, sitting and walking. It also illustrates how rests and changes of position can be built into the plan.

EXAMPLE: PACING AN INDIVIDUAL ACTIVITY – COOKING A MEAL

For standing tolerance of 15 minutes and sitting tolerance of 10 minutes – plan what you need: menu, ingredients, utensils needed, time, and allow for pacing of activity in this.

Collect ingredients together	*5 minutes standing/walking*
Rest	
Prepare vegetables	*10 minutes sitting*
Rest	
Cooking	*15 minutes standing – 1st stage*
Rest	
Cooking	*15 minutes standing – 2nd stage*
Rest	
Lay the table	*5 minutes walking/standing*
Dish up meal and eat	*10 minutes walking/standing/sitting*

This principle can be applied to any activity.

ACTIVITY: PACING AN ACTIVITY

Take an activity such as gardening, cleaning the car, or a household task and break it down into stages with rests and changes of position.

When pacing an activity the individual increases their baseline at their own pace. The increase can be on a daily or weekly or in some cases even monthly basis. If the baseline is increased daily it must be able to be maintained. It is no good making a large increase one week and then having to reduce the following week. This is just reinforcing the cycle of overactivity/underactivity again. If this does happen then the baseline and the rate of increase needs to be reassessed. To increase the baseline and maintain it, the baseline must be realistic. It should be set at an achievable level and fit in with the individual's lifestyle.

ADAPTATION OF THE ENVIRONMENT AND POSITIONING

Adaptation of the environment and correct positioning can reduce or minimize pain. Sitting is something people take for granted, yet poor posture, resulting from the way in which people sit and the type of chair used, can cause pain and discomfort. Simple adaptations might involve using a cushion in the small of the back or a high-density foam wedge under the seat cushion to facilitate a better sitting position. Often people do not look at their everyday environment: they take it for granted. Small alterations can sometimes make life easier and activities less painful; for example, equipment that is used frequently should be at waist level and items that are used less often should be stored on high or low shelves, thus eliminating unnecessary bending and reaching. Kneeling, sitting or squatting rather than bending down to look for items in drawers, cupboards or washing machine can also facilitate good ergonomic use of the body. Eliminating any unnecessary or sustained bending or reaching postures can promote good ergonomic working postures. This enables the individual to avoid exacerbation of their pain. Pacing and planning of the workload in conjunction with correct positioning and adaptation of the environment to suit the individual can all aid pain control in the work environment.

In some disorders such as rheumatoid arthritis, aids and adaptations may have to be issued and implemented – e.g. kitchen or writing equipment with modified handles to facilitate grip or extended handles to compensate for joint restriction. This section is not all-inclusive and is intended only as an overview of this area within the context of pain. Any book on ergonomics or occupational therapy will provide more information on this subject.

FITNESS AND EXERCISE

Chronic pain patients have a tendency to overdo activities. This can be the result of frustration, determination, guilt at not contributing to the household chores or being a wage earner. However this results in increased pain, which increases the need to rest to alleviate the pain. These swings of overactivity followed by underactivity lead to poor pain and life control. The rests or avoidance of certain activities lead to stiffness of joints, weakness of muscles and general unfitness.

Pain may result in the avoidance of movement and normal everyday activity. If something hurts there is a tendency to keep it still and not move it. In the short term this is effective and the correct strategy to use. After an acute injury the damaged area needs to be rested for a short time to allow healing to occur.

Effects of inactivity

In the long-term pain situation, rest and inactivity will exacerbate the pain problem. The normal healthy joint is surrounded by soft tissue, i.e. muscles, ligaments, joint capsule, cartilage, everything apart from the bones. These soft tissues remain healthy through movement. As the muscles are used, blood pumps through them to supply them with oxygen and carry the waste products away. This allows the muscle to stay healthy and work well. If the muscles are not used they become stiff and weak, tire easily and have poor endurance, and develop fibrous tissue rather than new muscle cells. This leads to an increase in stiffness and muscles that are difficult or painful to stretch.

Calcium may be lost from the bones through inactivity: 6 months of complete inactivity results in a loss of up to 40% of the calcium, and the structure of the bone becomes weakened.

During normal movement the synovial fluid lubricates the joint surfaces, keeping them supple and nourished. When the body is inactive the stabilizing ligaments around the joints become weaker and are easily sprained or torn. The joints themselves become stiff, due to lack of lubrication.

Other effects of inactivity are seen in the heart and blood circulation. The average unfit person has 40% less maximum efficiency of the heart and circulation than a fit person. Inactivity results in weak contractions of the heart, sluggish circulation and higher blood pressure; people may be more anaemic and there is a higher incidence of blood clots occurring in the calves and lungs. The immune system may also be affected. People are more prone to colds, flu and other diseases and they are more likely to contract bronchitis or pneumonia following a cold. Other areas affected by inactivity include the brain, which may lead to a change in behaviour; the patient will feel tired, less mentally alert, may be sleeping poorly, feels depressed and is less able to cope with stress. The bowels, balance and coordination, hormonal levels and the ageing processes are also affected. Inactivity is physically, mentally and spiritually debilitating.

These effects can be seen in normal, seemingly healthy members of the population if they are generally inactive – for example the 'couch potato'. There is a tendency to drive rather than walk, to sit and watch television, and to avoid exercise. In the presence of chronic pain the problems are often compounded and aggravated, because people tend to respond to pain by restricting their activities even further. Many of the physical problems faced by people with chronic pain are due to inactivity rather than the original cause of the pain. Even if it is not possible to remove the cause of the pain, if activity is increased many of the physical and emotional problems people suffer from are diminished.

Aims of exercise

The aims of exercise are to reverse the effects of inactivity. Exercise helps the body to function more normally. For instance if the pain sufferer has bowel problems or suffers from shortness of breath when walking, as the fitness level increases these problems will diminish. Exercise increases general activity levels, stamina, confidence, coordination and mobility.

People with chronic pain often feel that they are unable to exercise because it aggravates the pain, or they are worried that they might cause more damage or harm. When they try to exercise, they are able to do very little because they are unused to exercise. This is discouraging. They may feel uncomfortable afterwards, get out of breath and have sore, aching muscles. The key to increasing activity is to pace the exercise and build up gradually and slowly (see above).

Exercises are not dangerous if they are carried out correctly. To begin with, if someone has been inactive the muscles will be sore afterwards; this is a normal reaction. If an athlete stopped training for a time then went straight back into a competition they would have sore muscles. This pain is not harmful and cannot be avoided completely. It can be moderated or reduced by gradually increasing activity, just as an athlete does in their training. As a person gets fitter the aches and pains will decrease.

Benefits of exercise

Exercise improves suppleness, strength and stamina. It increases mobility and improves posture by stretching the tight soft tissues and the stiff joints. Muscle strength is improved and this increases the protection and support of the joints, e.g. stomach and back muscles. Stamina increases the endurance or staying power. Movement becomes easier and is able to be sustained for longer periods of time. Activity becomes less demanding and muscles less fatigued. Exercise helps maintain good posture and weight control, and can improve coordination. It also decreases pain information because when the body is exercised endorphins are released.

For example, when the elbow is knocked the individual will rub it vigorously. By doing, this the gate is closed to the pain messages. When pain is experienced other pain-relieving techniques like massage and heat may also help to ease it. As well as being very relaxing, the heat and massage sensations may help to block the pain messages. Exercise is another type of message (just like heat and massage). When people are in pain they automatically move (or exercise) – they may rock from foot to foot or tilt the pelvis backwards and forwards. Very few people feel that they want to stay absolutely still when they are in pain.

The second way that exercise helps to decrease the pain information is by increasing the production of the body's own natural pain-killing substances. When the body is exercised vigorously it produces natural chemicals (endorphins) similar to morphine. These endorphins give a feeling of well-being and people who exercise regularly 'feel good'. People who exercise intensively and are at a high level of fitness can become addicted to exercise and have withdrawal symptoms if they stop exercising; this is known as the 'runner's high'.

Fitness

Fitness means different things to different people. An athlete may only think himself fit if he can run a mile in under 4 minutes. Other people may feel they are fit if they can walk a mile at any speed, or do the gardening. Pain affects all areas of physical activity, including everyday things like getting out of the bath, or favourite hobbies. If activity is avoided for long periods of time, fitness will suffer, so that everyday activities become difficult to carry out.

Measuring fitness

There is no single measure of fitness; it depends on several elements and the main ones are strength, suppleness and stamina. **Strength** is the force a muscle can generate (carrying heavy shopping, pulling a rope in a tug-of-war). **Suppleness** is the range of movement in the muscles and joints (being able to stretch up to reach shelves, bending down to touch the toes). **Stamina** is the ability to repeat a muscular action over and over again and depends mainly on the cardiovascular system, i.e. the heart muscle, lungs and circulation, and its ability to transport food and oxygen to the muscles and carry waste products away from them.

Suppleness and strength can be improved by carrying out gentle stretching and strengthening exercises but to improve stamina a more challenging activity is required, e.g. swimming, brisk walking, and using an exercise bike or cycling. These types of activity are called **aerobic exercises**.

Aerobic exercise

The word 'aerobic' means the sustained rhythmic movement of large muscles, using oxygen for energy. In other words these are the types of activities that will get us 'puffing'. For example, walking up 13 flights of stairs will cause the heart to beat faster and the breathing rate to increase by the time the top flight is reached. The heart, lungs and circulation system have to work harder to cope with this extra work. Exercising in a similar way will help exercise the heart in a healthy way. To improve stamina aerobic exercise should be carried out for 20 minutes three times a week at an intensity of about 60–80% of the individual's maximum capacity.

The benefits of aerobic exercise are that it strengthens the heart and lungs, lowers blood pressure and can aid weight control. It may help prevent osteoporosis and other diseases such as diabetes. It can also act as a 'stress beater', decreasing muscular tension and enabling the individual to cope with stress. Because the body releases its own painkilling substances aerobic exercise can result in a feeling of well-being – the 'feel-good factor'.

Monitoring your progress

An easy way to monitor aerobic exercise is to use the pulse rate. This is taken at the radial or carotid pulse points and the number of beats per minute is recorded. The resting pulse is the number of heart beats in 1 minute while the body is at rest. During exercise, the heart has to work harder so the number of beats per minute (pulse rate) goes up. By taking the pulse during or just after exercising and comparing it with the resting pulse the level of work can be monitored.

ACTIVITY: TO WORK OUT A TRAINING PULSE ZONE

To find the resting pulse, place the index and middle finger above the wrist in line with the thumb. Press lightly and count the beats in 30 seconds, and then multiply this by 2. Now work out the individual exercise training pulse zone by working out the formula below.

- *$220 - (age + resting pulse) = pulse limit$*
- *Pulse limit $\times 0.6$ + resting pulse = training zone (lower limit)*
- *Pulse limit $\times 0.8$ + resting pulse = training zone(upper limit)*
- *My pulse training zone is. . . to. . .*

If the pulse rate is taken during or just after the exercise is finished and it falls somewhere between the lower and higher figure, then the exercise is aerobic and will gradually increase the individual's fitness level.

This method is not suitable for people who are on medication for high blood pressure as the heart rate is kept artificially low by the medication.

Before exercising, gentle movements should be used to warm up the body. There is less likelihood of strain if the body is warmed up first. Similarly, the body should be cooled down slowly following exercise. At the end of the aerobic activity the individual should be encouraged to walk around for a short while or do some gentle stretches until their pulse rate returns to normal.

Pacing

Start with gentle aerobic exercise at first and for just a couple of minutes. Then gradually build up the exercise time to around 20 minutes. Aerobic exercise should be moderately hard work but not completely exhausting. If the individual is too puffed to talk or whistle while exercising they are working too hard (this is called the talk test). Eventually the pulse rate will return to the resting rate more quickly following exercise, but most importantly stamina and energy will increase so that the individual is able to increase their daily activity levels. It is important to find an aerobic activity that is enjoyable, as the individual is more likely to continue with it on a regular basis.

The back school concept

Back schools were first started in the 1960s in Sweden (Hayne, 1987). Physiotherapists had found that routine physiotherapy with back pain patients had a limited success rate. They decided to try a more radical approach which would include fitness, modification of activities and education relating to care of the back. Their aims were to give patients the ability to cope with back problems by using ergonomic concepts to relieve and prevent pain, education and exercise. This programme would enable the patient to have a pain-free lifestyle within the limits of their condition.

Back schools first came to Britain in the 1970s and can be found in both the National Health Service (NHS) and in the private sector. Back schools are run on a therapeutic and prophylactic basis and today are often part of a broader total programme of back care (Hayne, 1987; Tanner, 1987). They are often run by physiotherapists but many now have a team approach. The team usually consists of a physiotherapist and occupational therapist. Length of attendance varies from one 3-hour session per week for 4 weeks to daily attendance for a fortnight. The interaction between patients and therapists enables the sessions to be tailored to the needs of the group. The ultimate goal is to return the patient to their normal lifestyle and to prevent a relapse. Patients are taught basic exercises to improve stamina, strength and suppleness. They are encouraged to practise good back care in relation to daily activities, work and social life and to recognize which activities should be modified or avoided so that they do not stress their backs. Many back schools or back education programmes teach basic relaxation skills as well as exercises.

COGNITIVE BEHAVIOURAL APPROACH

Cognitive psychology states that our understanding of the world is based on views and assumptions that are influenced by our culture, background, experience and family situation. Behaviour can be changed by looking at alternative strategies and adopting other attitudes.

The behavioural approach places more emphasis on the environment. It is based on the belief that some actions are rewarded and others result in punishment or deprivation. The learning and recognition of the results of our interaction with the environment can lead to more appropriate behavioural responses.

Beck (1987) said that behaviour and cognition were inter-related and used behavioural experiments in the form of tasks to treat his patients. These tasks were designed to challenge and test their negative thoughts. For example, to encourage patients to confront a particular situation they were set the task of keeping a diary to document their thoughts, feelings and actions. The cognitive behavioural approach is used successfully in pain management, and is usually operated on a group therapy basis (this is explored in greater detail in Chapter 8).

APPENDIX 7A: DEEP MUSCLE RELAXATION SCRIPT

Here is a list of muscles and instructions on how to tense them, looking particularly at the muscles that are tensed when we are stressed. After tensing and relaxing each muscle, take a deep diaphragmatic breath, getting rid of any remaining tension as you breathe out.

For the hands and forearms	Make a fist.
For the biceps	Bend your arms at the elbows and try to touch your wrists to your shoulders.
For the triceps (back of upper arms)	Straighten your arms as hard as you can.
For the shoulders	Shrug your shoulders as if trying to make them touch your ears.
For the neck	Arch your neck backwards.
For the forehead	Raise your eyebrows as if surprised.
For the brows and eyelids	Squeeze your eyes tightly shut.
For the jaw	Clench your teeth together.
For the tongue and throat	Push your tongue hard against the roof of your mouth.
For the chest	Take a deep breath and hold it and then release the breath slowly.
For the hips and back	Arch your back and clench your buttock muscles.
For the stomach	Tense your stomach as if someone were going to punch it.
For the legs	Straighten out your legs and point your feet away from you.

APPENDIX 7B: AUTOGENIC RELAXATION SCRIPT

Make yourself comfortable, lying or sitting, and take a deep diaphragmatic inhalation. Exhale gently and notice a feeling of relaxation. There is no need to move during autogenics unless you want to make yourself more comfortable. The aim is to unwind, allowing yourself to focus on the sensations of relaxation. The many phrases help you to do this. Repeat them to yourself three times, pausing after each repetition. Take your time, keeping your breathing regular, calm and relaxed.

I am at peace with myself and fully relaxed.

My right arm is heavy (if the patient is left handed you may want to start with the left side first).

My left arm is heavy.

My right leg is heavy.

My left leg is heavy.

My neck and shoulders are heavy.

Take a deep, full breath and unwind even further.

My right arm is warm.

My left arm is warm.

My neck and shoulders are warm.

My heartbeat is calm and regular.

My breathing is calm and regular.

My stomach is warm and calm.

My forehead is cool and calm.

Take some time to enjoy the sensations of relaxation.

I am refreshed and completely alert.

If you find that any of the phrases make you or the patient uncomfortable, simply use:

I feel calm and relaxed.

8 | Cognitive behavioural approach

HISTORY

Behaviourism is a school of psychology associated with Watson. He stated that learning consisted of a change in behaviour, which was measured in terms of the altered response to a stimulus. These ideas were taken further by Pavlov's experiments in **classical conditioning**, where the basic unit of learning was seen in terms of a stimulus–response association. Pavlov was a Russian physiologist who carried out experiments on salivation, a reflex response in the mouth to the presence of food, seen in dogs. In his experiments he conditioned the dogs to salivate initially on the presentation of food accompanied by the sound of a bell. Eventually the dogs would salivate on hearing the sound of the bell only, as they had learned to associate this sound with food. In classical conditioning the animal has no control over the events that are altering in its environment. During classical conditioning specific stimuli elicit behavioural responses from the subject.

Edward Thorndike (1874–1949) was one of the pioneers of American psychology and is famous for his 'puzzle box' with which he studied instrumental conditioning. A hungry cat was put into a box and food was placed outside the box where the cat could see but not reach it. The cat had to manipulate a latch that held the door in place to get out of the box. Escape from the box was contingent upon the animal's behaviour. Thorndike argued that learning only occurs if the action or response has an effect. Manipulation of the latch opened the door so that the cat could reach the food. He proposed the **law of effect**, which stated that if a response has a favourable consequence it will be learned. **Reinforcement** was seen as the process of strengthening this association between response and consequence and the **reinforcer** was the agent responsible for the reinforcement, e.g. food and escape.

Burrhus F. Skinner started his research in the 1930s and followed in the Thorndike tradition. The type of conditioning studied by Skinner is usually described as **operant conditioning**. In operant conditioning environmental change is brought about by the performance of a particular behaviour or set of behaviours. Skinner used positive and negative reinforcement to increase or decrease the performance of a behaviour. **Positive reinforcement** is the process of strengthening the association between the behaviour or operant and the positive reinforcer. **Negative reinforcement** is the process whereby the behaviour leads to the avoidance or removal of an unwanted or unpleasant stimulus. Both positive and negative reinforcement can lead to an increase in the frequency of the performance of a given behaviour that is being reinforced. Skinner also used procedures called **shaping, extinction** and **punishment** (see below).

These theorists did not believe that thoughts and ideas had any effect on the response of the animal and were only concerned with observable behaviour. Tolman disagreed with this and proposed a model of cognitive learning. He proposed that behaviour was governed by a purpose. Behaviour was not a stereotyped response to a stimulus: it was goal-directed. Tolman's model of learning is referred to as **cognitive**, i.e. it involves the storing of information or facts learned about the world, which were called **cognitions**. Tolman said that behaviour was purposeful and was dependent on learning, expectations and circumstances. The cognitive behavioural management of chronic pain is based on the theories and findings of these psychologists.

COGNITIVE THERAPY

Meichenbaum (1977) said that 'cognitive therapy is based on self instruction as a means of blocking negative thoughts'. Jacobson (1929) used this technique in stress management by using progressive muscle relaxation and imagery as a means of recognizing stress and counteracting or blocking it. Cognitive therapy places the emphasis on the individual regaining control over their life. It is based on the development of cognitive coping strategies. Melzack and Wall (1991) cite distraction and imagery as cognitive coping skills. Patients may be encouraged to use their imagination to reinterpret the pain or their subjective experience in terms other than pain.

BEHAVIOUR THERAPY

Behaviour therapy has its roots in classical conditioning and its aim is to extinguish learned behaviour patterns. Behaviour modification, using operant conditioning, offers positive rewards to establish or extinguish new behaviour. Treatment is based on the modification of inappropriate learning that has occurred in the past. Wolpe (Wolpe and Lange, 1964) used systematic desensitization with phobias. This used relaxation and progressive exposure to the stimulus causing the phobic response, and is called **extinction**. Other methods known as **flooding** were also used. The feared stimulus was confronted and this prevented avoidance behaviours from having a reinforcing effect. In some situations the patient may be accompanied by a therapist when undergoing this treatment. This is known as **modelling**, where the therapist acts as a role model in coping with the situation and can offer reassurance and advice. In chronic pain management some pain centres have a system where patients who have completed or are undergoing a course are used as role models with new patients. In this way the aims and concepts of the course are reinforced by people who have been active participants in the process and have found it useful in coping with pain.

In operant conditioning (see above), behaviour is changed by manipulating the consequences of an action through negative/positive reinforcement. Factors in the individual's environment that maintain behaviours are identified and these are then altered. In this way complex behaviour patterns can be modified by manipulating of rewards and punishments.

COGNITIVE MEDIATORS IN PAIN REDUCTION

Reese (1983) compared the effects of cognitive strategies, relaxation training and pharmaceutical placebos on tolerance for cold pressor pain. He found that they were all equally effective in enhancing the subject's expectation of pain relief. However, only the group using cognitive strategies showed any significant increase in pain tolerance. Bandura (1977, 1982) considered that **self-efficacy** helps to produce behavioural change. Self-efficacy involves the individual's expectations as to their ability to use coping strategies effectively. Marino, Gwynn and Spanos (1989) carried out experiments where the subject's expectations were manipulated in relation to their ability to use imagery and distraction techniques when a limb was immersed in icy water. They found that distraction techniques were as effective as imagery-based strategies and that the individual's perception of pain intensity was reduced. The same group of subjects reported a greater reduction in pain intensity when they used strategies associated with positive efficacy information and less reduction when the strategies were associated with negative efficacy information. The subject's expectations of how successful their efforts were likely to be modified their response to painful stimulation.

The role of distraction techniques

Distraction is when attention is focused on a stimulus other than the pain – e.g. reading, listening to music or watching television. Often, techniques using mental imagery or slow rhythmic breathing are used as a means of distraction. Distraction may increase pain tolerance and decrease the perceived intensity, as pain ceases to be the focus of attention. However, when the distraction stops pain becomes the central focus of the individual's awareness and is often accompanied by fatigue and irritability. There are many cited instances within sport of distraction, where athletes have sustained injury and continued to compete or play seemingly unaware of either pain or injury. Wynn Parry (1980), in his study on brachial plexus injuries, reports that patients who had severe pain found that their pain was reduced when they were absorbed in work. Many studies have been carried out on the effects of auditory input on pain. It has been found that a wide range of sound frequencies can be used to decrease pain, such as music and white noise. Melzack *et al.* (1980) found that distraction techniques were only effective if the pain intensity was constant or increased slowly. If the level of pain intensity rose sharply distraction techniques were not effective.

Assertiveness

Assertive behaviour is where the individual is able calmly, clearly and confidently to explain to others by their words or actions their preferred course of action. It also involves the individual taking the initiative for their actions. Assertiveness is a way of protecting one's own rights and needs without violating those of others (Keable, 1989). A lack of assertiveness may result in the patient bottling things up, being tense or resentful, avoiding confrontation and losing their temper. If the patient is assertive they are able to ask for help when they need it, they are able to say 'No' and ask for explanations when they don't understand the information they are given. Assertiveness means that the individual is able to make their feelings or worries known without causing an argument or becoming angry. They become more sociable and they are able to raise issues at the appropriate time. Rim and Masters (1974) stated that assertive behaviour is 'interpersonal behaviour involving the relatively direct expression of feeling in a socially appropriate manner'. Jakubowski-Spector (1973) said that assertiveness is 'a type of interpersonal behaviour in which a person stands up for their legitimate rights in such a way that the rights of others are not violated'. The aim of assertive behaviour is to enable the individual to communicate in a clear and confident manner without being aggressive.

COGNITIVE FACTORS IN PATIENTS' RESPONSE TO ILLNESS

Sensky (1990) states that the major influencing factors in patients' response to illness are their cognitions, i.e. their beliefs, thoughts and attitudes to illness. Emotional disturbances are associated with dysfunctional cognitions. 'Learning to identify and modify dysfunctional cognitions are core elements of cognitive therapy' (Beck and Emery, 1985). Martin *et al.* (1989) found that cognitive therapy was more effective with subjects who had high chronicity scores. Fordyce (1984) says that 'clinical pain, when seen from the perspective of a behavioural or learning /conditioning model, may lead to quite different inferences from those derived from a disease model'. **Operant learning** describes a process in which the frequency of occurrence of a given behaviour is modified by the consequences of it.

Operant principles in cognitive behaviour therapy

Therapy employing the principles of operant conditioning is used in the treatment of chronic pain patients. Operant conditioning is used to modify pain-related behaviour patterns through positive and negative reinforcement. This approach concentrates on the elimination of pain-related behaviour not on pain reduction. Pain-related behaviours may include verbalization of pain, avoidance of specific activities and the overuse of medication.

In operant conditioning learning is facilitated by the reinforcement of a particular behaviour, either negatively or positively. Any consequence (stimulus or event) of a given behaviour that is associated with an increase in the frequency of that behaviour or its maintenance is known as a **reinforcer**. The reinforcer is identified only by its apparent effect on the behaviour it follows.

Reinforcement schedules

A **schedule of reinforcement** describes the relationship between a given behaviour and a given reinforcer. There are two main types: **ratio schedules** and **interval schedules**. Ratio schedules involve reinforcers which are presented according to a given number of responses. This may be after one, two or more responses. For example the workers in a factory who do 'piece-work' are paid for every item they make, rather than for the number of hours they work. Interval schedules are where the reinforcer is presented according to a given time interval, providing a given response occurs in that period. For example, where the workforce are paid according to the number of hours they spend at work, they may only be paid provided that they carry out specified tasks or duties within that time.

In ratio and interval schedules the response can be fixed or variable. For example, in a ratio schedule there may be five responses in a fixed schedule and an average of five in a variable schedule, where reinforcement is given after two, six or seven responses. Similarly, in interval schedules, either a fixed or variable amount of time may be specified, e.g. 1 minute in a fixed schedule and an average of 2 minutes in a variable schedule.

Different patterns of behaviour are associated with different schedules of reinforcement. When a new behaviour is being learned a fixed ratio reinforcement is usually most effective, as it provides frequent and immediate reinforcement. Once the behaviour has been learned the frequency is usually greatest under a variable ratio schedule. If a fixed interval schedule is used, the response rate tends to be low for most of the interval, but increases rapidly towards the end of the interval – in, for example, the student who is given several weeks to prepare an essay and does all the work in the final week! A variable interval schedule is usually associated with a higher and more even rate of response than a fixed interval schedule. In the context of pain management, and the changing or modifying of behaviours, the schedule of reinforcement has important implications for the acquisition, maintenance and extinction of behaviours.

Reinforcement thinning

When a new behaviour is being learned regular and frequent reinforcement is needed. Once the behaviour has been learned its frequency will usually be greatest if intermittent reinforcements are given, the reinforcers being gradually withdrawn. Intermittent reinforcers (as, for example, in gambling) are the most powerful. Once the gambling habit has been learned, it is the possibility of winning next time that keeps the gambler hooked – to maintain the behaviour they only have to win occasionally. If they won every time they would get bored and the behaviour would diminish.

Discriminitive stimuli or cues

Discriminative stimuli or cues result in a given behaviour occurring and the consequence (i.e. reinforcer) that follows being predictable. This describes the relationship between a stimulus, a behaviour and a consequence. For example, a red traffic light tells the motorist to stop. If he ignores this, the likely consequence is an accident or a fine, both of which can be avoided by stopping. The traffic lights are acting as a discriminative stimulus. A discriminative stimulus in chronic pain could be an activity that increases or triggers the pain, e.g. hoovering or driving. Every time the activity is carried out pain is experienced; eventually the individual stops the activity so that the consequence of the activity, pain, is avoided.

Shaping

This is the reinforcing of successive approximations of a target behaviour until the target behaviour occurs. For example, when a child is learning to speak their efforts at communication are reinforced (i.e. with praise) whenever they make a sound that is near to the actual word. Reinforcement is then graduated so that it is only provided when the words uttered by the child are correct and then when they are able to string them together in a sentence or place them in the correct context. In other words, as the responses become nearer to the target ones, the criteria for reinforcement are gradually altered until reinforcement is only given when the desired or correct responses are made. Reinforcement is used in chronic pain management. Initially the patients will be praised for every attempt to modify behaviour or exercise (even if it is only at a very low level). As they improve in stamina and are able to cope with their pain, praise will only be given for goals that are achieved.

Generalization

There are two types of generalization: stimulus generalization and response generalization. **Stimulus generalization** is when a given behaviour, normally associated with one discriminative stimulus, occurs in the presence of similar stimuli or cues. As the stimuli become less similar to the original the given behaviour occurs less often – for example, the response when driving on the motorway to a car with a light on the top, which looks like a police car, versus someone in a car that could be a police car, versus someone in a car that clearly isn't a police car.

Response generalization is when a range of similar behaviours occur in the presence of a given discriminative stimulus; although the stimulus stays constant the behaviours may vary. For example, a partner might ask us to do the hoovering. Sometimes we do it immediately, sometimes after a delay, sometimes we do it well and sometimes poorly. If the partner responds with praise irrespective of when or how well the task is carried out we are unlikely to carry it out either immediately or well. But if we are praised only when we do it immediately and well, we are more likely to carry out the task in this way on future occasions (see Shaping, above).

Extinction

Extinction is the reduction of the frequency of a given behaviour to zero. This can be achieved by the removal of all reinforcers or by using an infrequent reinforcer. This is known as **straining the ration**. In the initial stages of the extinction process the response rate may increase in the short term before declining. For example, when a baby is put to bed the parent may let it cry rather than picking it up and rocking it. This will initially result in louder crying (known as an **extinction phenomenon**). However, this behaviour will eventually stop provided the reinforcer (picking up and cuddling/rocking) is not provided. Similarly, pain behaviour may increase in the short term when it is ignored but will eventually decline because it is not being positively reinforced by attention. The speed of extinction is determined mainly by the previous use of reinforcers. Rapid extinction can be achieved when the behaviour has previously been reinforced regularly at frequent intervals. Gradual extinction occurs when the behaviour has been reinforced intermittently.

APPLICATION OF COGNITIVE BEHAVIOURAL PRINCIPLES IN PAIN MANAGEMENT

Interdisciplinary pain teams use the cognitive behavioural approach in pain management with groups of both inpatients and outpatients. This approach uses education in relation to pain, posture and ergonomic principles, the teaching of coping strategies such as relaxation and exercise and the application of behavioural principles in pain management. 'The emphasis is on function and changes in quality of life caused by the pain, rather than on the underlying pathology' (Ralphs, 1995). The pain sufferer is shown how to deal with unhelpful beliefs about pain and reactions to pain (Kavanagh, 1995). The success of the treatment is not seen in terms of pain reduction. Improvement in quality of life, function and mood and the achievement of goals are the measures used in chronic pain management. The majority of programmes use a group format and are run on both an inpatient and outpatient basis.

Analysis of chronic pain behaviour

The behaviours seen in chronic pain may include a reduced level of functional or **well behaviours**, e.g. work, household chores, social activities, sport activities. There may be an increase in the frequency of motor pain behaviours such as limping, rubbing or tensing of the body. The individual may also complain about pain and other somatic symptoms, demonstrating an increase in verbal pain behaviour. They may also have increased their intake of analgesics, antidepressants and sedative/hypnotic medication, coffee, tea or alcohol. Many use aids such as walking sticks, braces, collars and corsets, make more frequent visits to their GP and have increased their use of health service facilities.

The reduction in the level of well behaviours is initiated by the onset of pain and is maintained by the avoidance of aversive consequences ('If I don't do this activity then the pain will not start/increase'). The patient comes to associate well behaviours with increases in pain intensity and so avoids them. The pain acts as a negative reinforcer for the avoidance of activities associated with well behaviours.

Increased levels of verbal and motor behaviour are maintained by positive reinforcement, such as the attention and concern that the individual receives from family and friends (Fordyce, 1976). The taking of medication for pain may be reinforced when it is followed by pain relief or sedation, and in the early stages this will work; however, as tolerance develops to the medication, the effects tend to diminish but pain reduction (due for instance to rest) may still be attributed to the medication. The patient is receiving an intermittent reinforcer, which establishes a strong pattern of behaviour so that there is a strong association between the taking of medication and pain relief.

The use of appliances and equipment may indicate a lack of confidence in relation to the individual's ability to walk or stand independently. It can also communicate to others that the user is disabled, thus lowering expectations of the patient and enabling them to avoid unwanted or difficult situations and tasks. As appliances and equipment tend to be a visible indication to others of a patient's problem they may feel that people will believe that they have pain if they use them. They often find that friends, family and the public help them more when they are using their sticks, collar, etc., so that the invalid behaviour is reinforced.

The use of medical facilities is reinforced by the medical profession, as complaints of pain are usually listened to and met by suggestions of further investigations or treatments. In contrast, attempts at 'well behaviours' may not be particularly noticed or reinforced. This reinforces the pain behaviour and encourages the continued use of medical services.

Behavioural management

The negative and positive reinforcers for reduced activity level and increased pain behaviours should be identified and well behaviours should be systematically reinforced, using positive reinforcers, so that there is an increase in them. At the same time any aversive consequences of increased activity should be minimized by, for example, increasing general stamina and fitness levels. Reinforcement of pain behaviours should be withdrawn by praising well behaviours and ignoring pain behaviours. Reinforcement of particular behaviours should be systematic and should be applied consistently by all the staff involved. Behaviour reinforcement should also comply with the principles of shaping, reinforcement thinning and extinction. Negative thoughts and beliefs should be challenged and restructured by the use of self-control principles and cognitive techniques.

Cognitive strategies are used to reduce the frequency of maladaptive and catastrophizing cognitions such as 'I can't go on' and 'Why won't somebody help me?' They are also used to establish the habit of self-reinforcement for well behaviours so that, when the patient is within the home environment, they are able to maintain their progress without the external reinforcement provided by staff or therapist. Operant conditioning methods are based on the assumption that even complex patterns of behaviour can be altered by the application of positive or negative reinforcement.

Pain programmes using the cognitive behavioural approach use various techniques and strategies. These techniques include relaxation, distraction, operant conditioning, exercise and fitness, activity analysis, problem solving and work evaluation. There is an emphasis on correct positioning of the body to carry out tasks, pacing, goal setting and on the fitness of the individual. At the same time the whole team applies an approach of positive reinforcement of well behaviours and negative reinforcement of sickness behaviours. Many pain programmes have a strong educational element, applied both to the functioning of the body and to how injury occurs and the correct postural use of the body when carrying out tasks. Some programmes encourage the patients to keep activity charts on which they set their goals and record their achievements. The charts can act as reinforcers and cues for self-reinforcement and behavioural change. The use of activity charts also increases the patient's independence and self-esteem as it is they, not the team, who control and set the goals for the activities. The patient is also encouraged to give themselves credit for their achievement (**self-attribution**), rather than crediting the therapist or team with their achievement. This is important for maintaining progress once the course or treatment programme is finished. The patient must learn to reinforce themselves for positive change; reinforcement might be a rest or an occasional treat. For example, some patients reward themselves with a biscuit or some chocolate. The aims of the cognitive behavioural approach in the pain management programme are to increase function, self-esteem, control of the pain and independence in social and physical activities, and to reduce the individual's stress and tension levels. The patient is an active participant in the programme, with the team members providing education and information and facilitating change within the context of pain management.

FURTHER READING

Lipchick, G., Milles, K. and Covington, C. (1993) The effects of multidisciplinary pain management on locus of control and pain beliefs in chronic non terminal pain. *Clin. J. Pain*, **19**, 49–57.

Loeser, J. D. and Egan, K. J. (1989) *Managing the Chronic Pain Patient: Theory and Practise at the University of Washington Pain Centre*, Raven Press, New York.

Pither, C. E. and Nicholas, M. K. (1991) Psychological approaches in chronic pain management. *Br. Med. Bull.*, **47**(3), 743–761.

Williams, D. and Keefe, F. (1991) Pain beliefs and the use of cognitive-behavioural coping strategies. *Pain*, **46**, 185–190.

Complementary therapies

The services of alternative or complementary therapy are being used more frequently in the last decade by the general public (Fulder and Munro, 1982). Studies carried out in the 1980s have shown that patients look for help with long-term, unresolved problems that the medical model seems unable to cope with, such as pain. Patients are often self-referred but many general practitioners (GPs) now recommend alternative practitioners or refer directly to them.

ACUPUNCTURE AND ACUPRESSURE

Acupuncture has been used for pain relief for many centuries but its effects in both acute and chronic pain are variable. The Chinese believe that good health is a state of energy balance within the body. They believe that the energy of life, the *chi,* consists of a balance between the opposites *yin* and *yang. Yin* is seen as negative, cold, dark, passive, hidden, female and solid, while *yang* is positive, warm, light, active, open, male and hollow. Both are seen as opposite ends of a continuous spectrum.

The aim of Chinese medicine is to correct any imbalance in these forces, since this is believed to be the cause of disharmony or disease, and to allow the body's healing mechanisms to work. The Chinese see disease as a symptom of an underlying energy imbalance.

The ancient Chinese observed that certain areas of the skin became more sensitive when a particular organ or function of the body was impaired. These areas are known as **points** and they are linked to the organs which they influence by pathways known as **meridians**. The energy of life flows along these pathways. There are 12 main meridians and two running down the front and back of the body. Points along each meridian affect not only the major organ associated with it, but also other parts of the body that relate to that organ. For example, disorders of the nose and throat can be treated through points on the lung meridian, because they are involved in breathing.

Aims and effects

The aim of acupuncture is to identify the imbalance of energy that is causing the disease and, by inserting very fine needles at sensitive points along a particular meridian or meridians, to stimulate or reduce the energy flow until the harmonious balance is restored.

Western medicine considers that acupuncture helps relieve pain and muscle tension by several mechanisms. These consist of local effects around the treatment point itself, the reflex nervous pathways between skin and muscle, the release of the body's pain-relieving hormones in the brain and spine and the blocking of pain transmission, either as it enters the spine or by preventing it from being relayed upwards to the brain.

Professor Ronald Melzack suggests that some chronic back pain may still occur after the original reason for the pain has ceased to exist because 'pain memories' have developed in the brain stem, rather like short-circuits in an electrical system. Professor Melzack suggests that one effect of acupuncture could be that it disrupts these short-circuits and effectively switches them off, so that pain relief persists even after the acupuncture stimulus has ceased.

Personality and the nature of pain

Many acupuncturists find that a good result from this type of treatment depends on the personality of the patient as well as the medical condition. Patients are classified as good responders and poor responders. A good responder does not apparently have to believe in the treatment. It has been found that they are usually decisive, impulsive, artistic or creative and ready to take risks. A poor responder is the opposite.

A study carried out in America showed that benefit from treatment also depends on the exact nature of the pain. The study consisted of 38 people suffering from low back pain. They were tested with spinal injections of increasing strengths. Those whose pain could be blocked by relatively weak injections benefited from acupuncture. After seven half-hour treatments their pain was reduced, on average, by 63% and the relief lasted for nearly 4 months. Those needing stronger solutions of anaesthetic and those whose pain was identified as having a psychological component did not benefit to the same extent from acupuncture. Other research has shown that benefit can be derived from treatment at non-acupuncture points as well as traditional acupuncture points. Some patients have shown benefit from simple dry needling of trigger points.

Professor Chang Hsiang-Tung of the research centre, the Institute of Physiology, in Shanghai stated that 'traditional Chinese acupuncture, like many other things, is not all perfect, consisting naturally of both pearls and rubbish' (Tanner, 1987).

Auricular acupuncture

Some acupuncturists treat only through points in the ear, since there is thought to be an entire system on each ear that represents all the organs and functions of the body. This is known as auricular acupuncture.

Moxibustion

Chinese- or Japanese-trained acupuncturists may use a smouldering moxa stick, cone of moxa or ball of moxa placed on the end of a needle or directly on the skin. The moxa (the leaf down of the plant *Artemesia moxa*) is removed when the sensation of heat is uncomfortable. It rarely burns the skin: sometimes a small blister occurs. When moxa is placed on the end of a needle, heat is conducted down the shaft and produces a pleasant sensation that relieves pain and relaxes taut muscles. It is said to clear the blocked channels, and the flow of *chi* energy is re-established.

Shiatsu or acupressure

Some acupuncturists treat without needles. Instead they massage the selected acupuncture points, especially if they are tender. Other practitioners use massage either before or after needling. The massage technique is different from the Western method, which is primarily designed to relax the muscles and stimulate blood circulation. The Eastern massage technique is used to stimulate points or entire meridians with finger pressure, elbow pressure, stamping, scratching and so on. Shiatsu is currently used in the treatment of cancer and AIDS. Acupressure is thought by Western scientists to release enkephalins after 5–10 minutes of treatment, when the patient starts to feel some relief from the pain. The effect of the treatment may last up to 30 minutes following treatment.

Advances in acupuncture

New equipment in acupuncture does not involve the use of needles. The electro-acupuncture kit works by detecting the acupuncture points, by finding areas that will conduct a current more easily. These areas are stimulated electrically using a probe that does not penetrate the skin. However, it has been shown that, if you rub a metal probe over the skin anywhere, you will eventually sensitize a small area, allowing a current to pass. Laser acupuncture, it is claimed, will fire a laser beam through a target area of skin and the treatment is completed in a few seconds without pricking the skin. This method of treatment, when carried out under experimental conditions, has not proved to be as effective as traditional acupuncture methods.

ALEXANDER TECHNIQUE

The Alexander technique increases awareness of balance, posture and movement in everyday activities. This can bring into consciousness tensions previously unnoticed, and helps to differentiate between appropriate and inappropriate tensions and effort. This technique is based on the principle of relaxing muscles, particularly the neck and shoulder muscles, and adopting a posture that puts the least amount of stress on the spine.

This technique was developed in the late 19th century by an Australian actor, F. Matthias Alexander. Following temporary retirement from an acting career due to a sudden loss of voice during performance, he diagnosed his own problem, as doctors were unable to help him. He found that, just before delivering any speech on stage, he pulled his head backwards and downwards in a manner which cut off his voice. Following this discovery he went on to form the **Alexander principle**. His approach differed from osteopathy and chiropractic in that he did not regard vertebral malalignment or a reduction in mobility as problems to be tackled in isolation. He believed that they were due primarily to misuse and maintained that habit and use dictate function. Posture exerts a constant influence on general function, physiologically and psychologically. We all have a unique posture, just as our fingerprints and voiceprints are also unique. Because of this the Alexander technique is usually taught on a one-to-one basis. All pupils are taught techniques developed specifically for their own posture, which they then practise daily. The course may involve just five or six lessons over a few weeks, or it can last up to a year.

Technique

The teacher works with the individual in a sitting, standing or lying position, depending on the requirements of the individual. People who have learned the Alexander method commonly say that it is a question of undoing all the habits that have become second nature. Often one is asked to adopt postures and positions that feel unnatural because bad posture has grown to feel more natural than good posture. The student relearns habits of movement through the repetition of basic movements until they are able to do them automatically. This technique is especially useful for the avoidance of postural pain. The emphasis is placed on postures being relaxed as this ensures ease of movement and diminishes the stress and strain on the joints. Sarah Barker (1978) defined Alexander's key concept of use as follows: 'Good use means moving the body with maximum balance and coordination of all parts so that only the effort absolutely needed is expended'.

AROMATHERAPY

Aromatherapy covers any treatment using the aromatic oils obtained from a variety of plants for their medicinal properties. The 'essential oils' are extracted by water extraction, heat treatment or oil basing. They can be used in their pure form (this is very potent) or diluted using a carrier oil. The pure oils can be taken internally in drop form and this method of treatment is used extensively on the Continent. The pure oil should only be taken on the advice of a qualified and experienced practitioner.

The commonest way of using oils is in a dilute form. The diluted oil is mixed with a base or carrier oil and this is then added to bath water. When the aromatic oils are used for massage they are diluted further in oil.

Different plants have different properties: for example rosemary (*Rosmarinus officinalis*) is used for stimulation and sweet marjoram (*Origanum majorana*) is considered to have a relaxing effect. Essential oils are used to calm the nerves, stimulate digestion and aid depression. One of the most active properties in the oil is its aroma. The quickest path to the brain is via smell and the smell association area in the brain is located next to the area for memory. This is why different scents can conjure up memories and evoke feelings from the past. This also explains why aromatherapy treatments can affect or change the mood of the individual.

Massage is often used as a form of treatment by aromatherapists. Many of the oils have specific therapeutic actions including pain relief. Some oils are relaxing (*Lavandula angustifolia*, *Lavandula officinale* (lavender), *Jasminum officinale* (jasmine), *Rosa damascena* (rose)) whereas others can be used for muscle pain as they have a local warming effect (*Juniperus communis* (juniper), *Piper nigrum* (pepper)). Aromatherapy can also aid relaxation and is used with patients who have sleep problems. In a vaporized form the oils may be used for sinusitis and insomnia.

Oils should never be taken internally without the advice and monitoring of a qualified practitioner. Many oils can be used safely at home, but pure oils should always be diluted in a carrier first before applying to the skin in case they cause burning. Pure oils can be added to bath water or burned as a room scent. When using in this way, always follow the instructions on the bottle, as some bath oils contain essential oils in diluted form.

Essential oils vary in price depending on the availability of the plant. For example, jasmine is very expensive because only a small amount of oil can be obtained from each plant. Rosemary, on the other hand, is relatively inexpensive as the plant is widely available and yields more oil.

Many nurses and occupational therapists are now training as aromatherapists. They use their skills predominantly in the fields of geriatrics, terminal care, pain relief and, more recently, with HIV/AIDS patients. Aromatherapists can also be found in alternative health-care clinics, fitness centres and beauty salons in the private sector.

HOMOEOPATHY

Homoeopathic medicine is based on the principle that 'like cures like'. In the 18th century a German doctor, Hahnemann, noticed that certain natural drugs derived from plants and chemicals reproduced the symptoms of certain diseases if they were given to healthy people. He discovered that these same drugs cured the diseases whose symptoms they reproduced. Hahnemann carried out further investigations and discovered that more dilute mixtures were more potent than concentrated mixtures. When homoeopathic drugs are administered they are always given in very dilute doses. Because of this dilution homeopaths argue that their treatment is much safer and freer from side effects than conventional medicine. Remedies can be given as tablets, liquids, powders or ointments.

Remedies work by stimulating the body's natural defence system. There are a wide variety of homoeopathic drugs to treat a single condition, each suited to a particular type of person, unlike conventional medicine, where there is one drug or group of drugs for each condition. Homoeopaths treat on the basis of the patient's psychological and physiological constitution. There are several home-opathic hospitals in the country and some GPs have homoeopathic training. Many chemists now stock homoeopathic remedies, which can be bought with-out a prescription.

HYPNOTHERAPY

Hypnosis is a trance-like state in which the subject's attention is focused on the hypnotist. In this state, attention to other stimuli is diminished through the manipulation of attention and the use of suggestion. Many patients have found that hypnotherapy can help to control their pain. Under hypnosis, the control over the conscious mind is suspended temporarily, so that the individual's subconscious thoughts, feelings and memories can be reached. Through hypnotherapy access can be gained to subconscious functions in the brain such as the translation of messages from the nervous system into feelings of pain. In this way the individual can gain control over their perception of pain. The most suitable patients for this type of therapy are those who are able to trust others and relax. If the individual does not respond effectively to hypnotherapy, self-hypnosis techniques can sometimes be taught. This technique is a form of auto-suggestion, but needs to be learned from a qualified hypnotherapist or psychologist. The aim is to achieve physical and mental relaxation so that the mind is receptive to new concepts.

A study of hypnotherapy and chronic back pain, undertaken in San Francisco in 1977, was carried out with eight people who had all been in pain for between 1 and 23 years. They were given between 8 and 14 hourly sessions of hypnosis. Initially they were all given relaxation training to reduce their muscular tension and increase body awareness. This was reinforced by further instructions in self-awareness, combined with breathing exercises (Tanner, 1987).

The aim of the hypnosis sessions was to show the patients how to reduce the pain by producing thoughts, images or feelings that were incompatible with it. For example, a patient might imagine an ice-pack being placed over or around the burning sensation of pain. Using this technique the patients were trained to raise or lower the pain level, proving the extent of their pain control. Once one painful sensation had been eliminated they would move on to the next aspect, such as throbbing, stabbing or twisting, and tackle it in the same way.

Finally, each person was taught how to extend their learning to control the level of pain in a wide variety of situations when fully conscious. When followed up 4 months after therapy, their pain was still reduced, they were sleeping better and enjoyed a more active social life. General levels of depression and anxiety had improved as a consequence. Consumption of painkillers was also reduced.

MASSAGE

Massage is an ancient treatment that can be traced back the ancient civilizations of China, India, Greece and Rome. Grant (1993) defines it as 'the treatment of muscles using rubbing or kneading'. It can aid suppleness by breaking down fluid retention and fatty deposits and releasing areas of immobility. It has also been used to aid relaxation, increase the circulation and relieve pain. However, massage will not relieve pain due to inflammatory disease. Massage is a natural extension of touch; as Calvert (1992) said, 'touch is the basis of all hands on therapies'.

Massage is usually carried out using cream or oil, which is massaged into the body using a range of techniques such as stroking, percussion, kneading and pummelling. There are various specialized massages such as sports or remedial massage, relaxation and skin massage.

Techniques vary and some therapists will move only the skin with light repetitious movements whereas others use a vigorous massage of the deep structures. When used as a treatment for pain the massage may be given at the pain site or distal to the pain. Ice massage may be used and this has a similar effect to acupuncture or TENS. Melzack, Guite and Gonshor (1980) gave patients with acute dental pain ice massage on the back of the hand on the same side as the pain. Pain intensity was decreased by 50%. They carried out similar experiments using ice massage on the opposite side of the body, which also gave significant pain relief.

Superficial massage is usually given to the back and shoulders using aromatic oils (see Aromatherapy, above). Other massages used include **retrograde massage**, which is used in acute hand injuries to assist blood and lymphatic flow. This is usually followed by active movement. **Pressure massage** is where the acupuncture or trigger points related to the pain are massaged with pressure. Pain relief is felt after the pressure is released. The pressure is thought to decrease the irritability of the trigger points. **Energy massage** can help pain, migraine, asthma and depression. This type of massage is more health- and less illness-focused than structural massage techniques. It is based on Norwegian physiotherapy technique and includes postural integration and biodynamics.

The aims of massage are to alleviate dysfunction and maximize function and to relieve pain. Massage can also aid relaxation, lymphatic drainage and improve the circulation.

OSTEOPATHY

Osteopathy was started in 1874 by Andrew Taylor Still, a doctor in Missouri, USA. He started schools in the USA and in 1917 the British School of Osteopathy was founded in London by one of his pupils, Dr J. Martin Littlejohn. There is also the British College of Naturopathy and Osteopathy in London, and the European College of Osteopathy in Maidstone, Kent. These colleges all have 4-year full-time diploma courses.

The osteopath concentrates on function and sees spinal disorders as abnormal movement of the joints. Osteopaths use leverage rather than thrusting movements and use massage-like techniques to stretch ligaments around the joint to restore the range of movement. Some osteopaths use gentle release techniques to ease away stress in tissues. When examining a patient, they employ a system of detailed palpation during diagnosis.

Osteopaths are trained to assess the structural integrity of the spine and other joints of the body. They do this through observing movement restrictions and areas of immobility and through palpation or touch.

CHIROPRACTIC

This is a form of manipulative therapy. Chiropractic was founded by a Canadian, Daniel David Palmer, in 1895. Chiropractors work in a similar way to osteopaths. However, they are distinct from osteopaths in that they rely on X-rays for diagnosis, and see problems in terms of the structure of the spine. Thrusting techniques are used to reposition specific bones to relieve disorders such as neck pain, back pain and headaches. The British Chiropractors' Association was established in 1925 and has a register of graduates from recognized colleges of chiropractic.

Applied kinesiology

The technique of applied kinesiology was originated by an American chiropractor, Dr George Goodheart, in 1965 and now forms a part of many chiropractic treatments. It is a system of muscle testing, the results of which are said to point to any deficiencies in organ function and general health. It was devised to correct structural imbalances and as an aid to diagnosis.

McTimoney technique

Another branch of chiropractic, called the McTimoney technique, is more recent. This concentrates on a wider approach to manipulation incorporating some chiropractic techniques with osteopathic concepts to develop a gentle form of bodywork.

CRANIO-SACRAL THERAPY

Cranio-sacral therapy and cranial osteopathy are used for the treatment of the whole body and to effect structural change. The techniques often involve direct contact with the patient's energy field. A gentler form is used in the treatment of newborn babies, the elderly and pain sufferers. This technique was developed in the 1900s by William Sutherland, an American osteopath. The hands are used to feel the individual's intrinsic movement patterns and the techniques used by the therapist amplify these patterns and establish the body's natural balance.

Sutherland found that there were links between areas of the body, and his theory was that the positioning of the skull bones could affect other parts of the body. He found that by limiting movement of specific cranial bones he could affect various parts of the body or cause emotional reactions. This was developed further by Dr Randolph Stone in the 1960s and Dr John Upledger in the 1970s, who developed the technique into a whole-body approach. This type of treatment is relaxing and increases the individual's body awareness. It is used for bringing about structural changes and has been beneficial in the treatment of health difficulties related to the birth process, such as forceps or suction techniques during the birth. Cranio-sacral therapists are usually osteopaths who have a postgraduate training in cranio-sacral techniques.

The spaces (**fontanelles**) between the skull bones, which are present at birth, disappear as the bones grow together but the skull bones retain the potential for mobility throughout life. Therapists believe that by the alteration of internal pressure, movement and release of energy the individual can increase their body awareness. The main source of inner motion is the production and reabsorption of cerebrospinal fluid. Movement is perceived through touch, and the rhythm and patterns of the movement act as indicators of the body's condition or state of well-being.

REFLEXOLOGY

Reflexology is based on the principle that there are reflexes in the feet which relate to all other parts of the body. Small pressure movements are used over both surfaces of the foot and around the ankle. The aim is to stimulate or relieve specific areas as well as to create overall change in the body. The areas of the body in need of treatment are usually felt in the foot as areas sensitive to the therapist's touch. The therapist is trained to feel tissue change relating to texture and tone. This type of treatment has a relaxing effect on the patient and can be used as a specific tool for relaxation and pain relief. Areas of sensitivity are indications of imbalance in the related part of the body. The movements of the reflexologist follow a 'map' which relates parts of the body to corresponding reflex points on each foot.

There are many other alternative philosophies, but the ones I have outlined are those most commonly sought or used by patients in pain. Some of these may be available under the National Health Service in some areas. The suggested reading at the end of this section is not all-embracing. There are many books and articles available at the current time and the following are meant as an introduction to or outline reading for the alternative philosophies.

FURTHER READING

Alexander, F. M. (1992) *The Use of Self*, E. P. Dutton, New York (Centreline paperback, 1986).

Grant, B. (1993) *A–Z of Natural Healthcare*, Optima, London.

Lockie, A. (1990) *The Family Guide to Homeopathy*, Hamish Hamilton, London.

Moore, S. (1988) *Chiropractic*, Optima, London.

Sandler, S. (1987) *Osteopathy*, Optima, London.

Tanner, J. (1987) *Beating Back Pain*, British Holistic Medical Association, Dorling Kindersley, London.

Tisserand, R. (1990) *The Art of Aromatherapy*, C. W. Daniel, Saffron Walden.

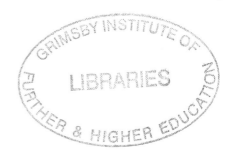

| 10 | **The role of professionals** |

Many health professionals are involved in the care of patients who have acute and chronic pain. They may work on a one-to-one basis or in the group setting, where they form part of an interdisciplinary or multidisciplinary team. Many health professionals may be involved in the care of the patient, for example the pain consultant, orthopaedic consultant, rheumatologist, general practitioner, specialist nurse, district nurse, occupational therapist, physiotherapist, psychologist, pharmacologist, dietitian, radiologist, social worker and ward staff. The care usually covers both the community and the hospital environment but for the purposes of this book will primarily be restricted to the hospital environment and the core team professionals. This chapter will cover the roles of the doctor, specialist nurse, occupational therapist, physiotherapist and psychologist – the pain team, practical advice on pain management programmes and guidelines for chronic and acute pain management.

THE DOCTOR

The consultant plays an important part in screening the patient to ensure that there is no underlying cause for the pain that can be treated or alleviated under the medical model of treatment. Consultants have access to all the relevant diagnostic tools, such as X-rays, MRI scans, blood tests and their own diagnostic skills (Chapter 5). Having determined that the patient's pain is not improved by medication, injections, surgery or other means such as physiotherapy or acupuncture, the consultant may refer to the pain team. The consultant usually has a good working knowledge of the concepts underlying the team's approach and will participate in the group programme. Depending on the consultant this participation will vary. Some consultants attend each group session and are available for patients to talk to on an informal basis. Others may attend only for specific lectures. The subjects usually covered by their talks within the group format can be divided into three areas: anatomy and structure of the spine, medication and disabusing the medical model.

Anatomy

The talk on anatomy and structure of the spine primarily covers the spine and the function of its relevant parts and will usually include the causes of back pain, the relevance of surgery and an explanation of diagnostic techniques that patients have undergone. This allows patients to air dissatisfaction with treatment and have their questions relating to treatment and diagnosis answered in informal surroundings away from the clinical setting of the consultation room. The emphasis of the consultant is on the fact that surgery can, in fact, make things worse and on the limitations of surgery. Patients usually find this talk informative and helpful in coming to terms with their problem.

Medication

The talk on medication acts as an endorsement of the pain team approach from a medical viewpoint. The aim of this discussion is to give information relating to the use and abuse of medication. The patients are encouraged to participate by listing the drugs they are currently taking. The consultant then discusses the use and side effects of the drugs and the dangers of long-term usage. The main points incorporated into this talk may be that drugs cease to be effective over time as the body becomes used to them; the fact that it is dangerous to increase the dosage because the drug doesn't seem to be having an effect, and the possibility of side effects due to high doses, such as confusion and muddled thinking; the dangers of drug dependency and the benefits of utilizing the patient's own skills in pain management.

Disabusing the medical model

Disabusing the medical model covers the concept that medicine is limited in terms of its ability to diagnose, cure and even manage chronic pain. In other words it is not infallible. The talk reinforces the concept of self-help. It also makes the point that doctors have problems dealing with chronic pain just as the patient does and that doctors too get frustrated because they are unable to 'cure' the patient. The patient may feel that their doctor does not have time for them or that the doctor thinks that they are malingering. This is not usually the case; the doctor is simply frustrated at not knowing what help or advice to offer next when all the standard treatments or advice have had no effect on the pain.

Doctors are trained to diagnose and treat health problems. When the patient goes to see a doctor this is what the doctor is hoping to do. This approach works well for short-term or acute problems but for long-term or chronic problems, which do not lend themselves to a specific diagnosis or cure, it does not work. Long-term problems require management strategies. Many doctors recognize this and, while they may not be able to offer any treatment, they allow time for the patient to sit and discuss their problems. This can act as a facilitating process for the patient to problem-solve and manage their pain.

The consultant is able to reinforce education about current theories of pain and the rationale of the various treatments, enabling the patient to appreciate the complexity of the problem. They also have a chance to ask questions about their particular histories, to express some of their disappointment and frustrations with past treatment and to readjust some unrealistic expectations of medical practice.

THE SPECIALIST NURSE

The clinical nurse specialist has a role to play in the clinical, educational and research field. There is no set standard for the specialist nurse in the pain field at the current time and most of their education, as with physiotherapists and occupational therapists, comes from colleagues working in the same speciality and from study days and conferences.

In the acute pain setting

The nurse is involved pre- and postoperatively with the patients and may carry out ongoing pain assessment as part of the care plan. In the preoperative assessment the nurse has the opportunity to alleviate anxiety and to ascertain any coping strategies the patient uses and their previous experience and expectations of pain. Ongoing evaluation and assessment of medication is an integral part of pain management in the acute setting. Other techniques the nurse may be involved with are TNS, nerve blocks, epidurals and spinal analgesia. Pain relief in the acute setting now has a higher priority than in the past. As nurses spend more time than other primary-care team members with the patients, they are ideally suited to monitor and manage pain on a daily basis.

The nurse plays an important role in the identification of pain and pain management. 'Pain is a bond between nurse and patient. Pain management is a pact between them. . . .How they work out pain management agreeable to both is the essence of good nursing care' (Copp, 1985). Although focusing on the management of pain, the nurse plays an important role in anticipating and preventing pain. Nursing interventions can be divided into three broad categories: firstly, teaching activities to enhance the patient's understanding of the significance and meaning of pain; secondly, using measures to alter the sensory input of the patient's perception of pain; and thirdly, helping the patient to develop skills in the self-management of pain.

The nurse has an important role to play in the identification of the patient's experience and perception of pain, facilitating communication with other team members and encouraging patient participation in the decision-making process.

Within the pain team environment

The nurse's role in the pain team is primarily that of helping chronic pain patients to reduce medication, acting as a link person between the consultant's clinics and the pain team, participating in the initial team assessment and, in some instances, running a seperate TNS clinic. The role varies between hospitals but the above are the predominant areas that the nurse covers. In some hospitals the nurse will teach relaxation and coping strategies for patients who have problems with sleep.

Coordinator

The nurse's role as a coordinator between the clinic and the team is very important. When the patients come for their team assessment the nurse is able to provide information about the patient's problems and relate some of the background history to the team. When the patient arrives for assessment they see a familiar face and this helps them to relax and participate more fully in the assessment. It also helps the consultant when a patient who has undergone a course is referred back to his clinic. The nurse is able to feed in information about the patient's progress or otherwise during the course, level of attendance and willingness to take the concepts of pain management on board. This two-way communication role, between the consultant and the pain team, is important in maintaining unity and exchange of information between the two areas.

Assessment

The nursing assessment may consist of levels of medication, use of pain charts and previous medical history. This is similar to some of the pain assessments carried out by nurses working with inpatients. Sometimes the nurse will carry out assessments such as the McGill Pain Questionnaire and the Hospital Anxiety and Depression Scores in the clinic with the patient prior to seeing the consultant. The nurse is also well qualified to explain different procedures to the patient, such as the assessment procedure by the pain team and day surgery procedures.

Medication

Research has shown that opiates, antidepressants and tranquillizers are unhelpful in chronic pain. They are often ineffective and can cause unwanted side effects such as drowsiness, dry mouth, constipation, memory problems and lack of concentration. Since the medication does not abolish the pain, nor enable patients to return to their previous level of function, the advantages and disadvantages of taking medication are discussed with the patient by the nurse. The nurse gives guidance on gradual reduction of medication. There are various methods of reduction. Some patients may continue taking their own tablets, but regularly, according to the clock (**time-contingent**), rather than when the pain is bad (**pain-contingent**). They are then encouraged to reduce their medication gradually on a planned schedule after discussion with the nurse. Others may reduce their medication using a cocktail, in which the active ingredients in liquid form are gradually reduced while the volume remains the same. Again this is taken according to time, not pain. Some patients may try using a TNS machine instead of medication. This is used on a planned basis: the TNS is substituted for medication and then the use of TNS is reduced. Again this is used on a time-contingent instead of pain-contingent basis. Patients are also encouraged to use other coping strategies, such as relaxation, instead of medication.

THE OCCUPATIONAL THERAPIST

Occupational therapy is 'the treatment of illness or disability through analysis and use of the occupations which fill up a person's time and space and engage the individual in activity' (Reed and Sanderson, 1983). As Pedretti and Zoltan (1990) say, occupational therapists utilize selected tasks to restore, reinforce and enhance performance. They facilitate the learning of new skills and techniques which are necessary for work, daily living or the correction of dysfunction. Treatment methods may include self-care assessment and training, orthotics, hand therapy, relaxation, the use of adaptive equipment, home evaluation and adaptation, work modification and energy conservation, and work retraining. Occupational therapists work with people of all ages in the physical and psychiatric sectors of the health service and in the community, where they may be based in special schools, social service departments or health centres.

Outpatient occupational therapist

Patients are seen for treatment of hand and arm injuries resulting in pain and in some cases lower limb injuries. Other patients who suffer pain may be referred from the orthopaedic consultant, rheumatology consultant and plastic surgeons. Following initial assessment and consultation with the patient about their problems and difficulties a treatment programme will be arranged. This generally includes activities to increase range of movement and function, desensitization, reduction of oedema and pain. Splints and pain management strategies may also be used. The strategies which can be used for pain management are goal setting, pacing, relaxation and a cognitive behavioural approach. Therapists should explain the aims of treatment and be prepared to discuss the patient's condition with them as this helps to reduce anxiety and stress levels. The activities used in the treatment programme will be dependent on the specific disorder and the individual needs of the patient.

Inpatient occupational therapist

When pain patients are seen as inpatients the treatment programme may include assessment for adaptation to seating, assessment of activities of daily living, feeding and writing adaptations and a domiciliary visit to the patient's home to assess the patient's independence in the home setting. Within this programme education on posture and pain management using pacing and relaxation may also be used. Patients seen as inpatients may include postoperative back or neck patients, patients with thalamic pain, terminal cases of cancer, rheumatology patients, patients suffering from motor neurone disease or multiple sclerosis, HIV sufferers, cardiac patients and amputees.

Occupational therapy in pain clinics

Many pain clinics only have a part time occupational therapist and other pain clinics may not have a specific occupational therapist working with them. In the latter situation patients are usually referred direct to the outpatient occupational therapy department.

Most of the occupational therapists working within the pain clinic setting are working to a cognitive behavioural model. The aims of the therapist are to encourage the patient to live as normal a life as possible, to facilitate functional independence in everyday activities and to encourage the patient to set realistic goals and pace their activities. The occupational therapist will assess the patient using an interview, assessment activities and written assessment forms. These usually relate to level of activity, previous history relating to both medical and work history, the onset of pain and type of pain, and the effect that the patient feels this has on their lifestyle and activity levels. In acute and chronic pain management the assessment of function highlights areas of dysfunction and enables the therapist to plan and discuss with the patient which coping strategies or interventions will increase their function or level of activity.

The occupational therapist looks at posture in relation to pain, seating and working positions and gives general advice on ways to overcome practical problems such as bathing, ironing, gardening, etc. The patients are encouraged to think positively and to set goals for themselves so that, where possible, they can lead the life they want to lead and not one that is ruled by their pain. Occupational therapists working within the pain clinic setting are working in an interdisciplinary or multidisciplinary team where patient treatment is group-orientated.

Specialist equipment

Specialist equipment is only issued when its use will help the patient to regain control over the practical aspects of their lives. For example, if the use of a bath board enables the patient to bath unaided then it helps the patient to regain control over their life. If the bath board enables a carer or family member to bathe the patient more easily, the invalid role is reinforced. The occupational therapist is often used as a resource on specialist equipment. The therapist's role may include the provision of information relating to equipment so that the patient can make an informed choice when buying equipment to facilitate independence.

Educating/facilitating role

The occupational therapist's role is an educating/facilitating one. The emphasis is on changing the environment to suit the individual and not *vice versa*. There is encouragement of postural awareness and how the body is used during activity. In line with the cognitive behavioural approach, activity is related to goal-setting and pacing. The occupational therapist has an advisory/facilitating approach rather than 'hands-on'.

THE PHYSIOTHERAPIST

Traditionally, physiotherapists work with patients using an approach based on a musculoskeletal assessment. A wide variety of treatment modalities are used, such as electrotherapy (including ultrasound, megapulse and, more recently, lasers). Other treatment methods may include exercise and manual therapy, or what is often described as 'hands-on therapy'. Historically, physiotherapy has always been a very tactile profession. Many of these conventional physiotherapy treatments involve the patient being the passive recipient, with the physiotherapist controlling the treatment.

Outpatient physiotherapy

In the outpatient department the pain patient will have a clinical examination by the physiotherapist and an interview in relation to previous medical history, the pain history – onset, what affects the pain, and type of pain – and the effect the pain or injury is having on the patient's lifestyle. The patient may be referred from general practitioners, consultants or other hospital departments. The treatment will vary according to current thinking and practice and the therapist themselves. The approach is usually one of the patient in the passive role with the therapist carrying out the treatment on them.

Physiotherapy in the pain clinic

Physiotherapists have been involved in working with pain clinics since the 1970s. Initially, this was less direct as the patients were referred from the clinic and treatments included ultrasound, TENS, back education and hydrotherapy. Now physiotherapists attend the consultant's clinic, receiving referrals direct from it. Others will work with a team of other professionals in a multidisciplinary setting. In this case they may spend part of their time working in the outpatient department as a specialist physiotherapist in pain management, seeing individual patients with pain problems. Their approach tends to be from a cognitive behavioural stance using the chronic pain model. The patient is expected to take an active participative role in treatment and the aim is for the patient to take responsibility for themselves and to have control over their lives instead of the pain controlling their activities.

After the physiotherapist has assessed the patient and the level of intervention is agreed with the rest of the team the patient may attend an outpatient pain management programme. The physiotherapist is involved with all areas of exercise and activity. The patients are given guidance on setting realistic achievable targets in relation to exercise and activity. Many chronic pain patients may have a negative view of physiotherapy intervention as in the past treatment may have made their condition worse. The approach used within the group setting helps to alleviate this as the patients are in control of their activities and monitor their own progress. The exercise may take the form of a group exercise session or individual fitness activity. The patient may need help from the physiotherapist in monitoring and modifying the exercise programme. Pain is not seen as a reason for stopping exercise. Pain behaviour is ignored and well behaviour reinforced. As patients understand more about the complexity of the pain experience, they are able to accept that 'hurt does not necessarily mean harm'.

Patients are encouraged to improve their mobility and exercise tolerance levels, their range of movement and ultimately their levels of fitness; to increase their understanding of good body posture and mechanics; and to challenge existing ways of carrying out activities. They are also shown how to maintain or improve these levels once they are achieved, with a maintenance programme.

The physiotherapist helps the patient to identify problems within all areas of activity. A functionally directed interview and simple physical activity tests are the tools of assessment. The physiotherapist is a facilitator, with the patient taking the active role in working towards improving levels of exercise and fitness activity. This is achieved by helping the patient to relearn the goal-setting approach and pacing of activity.

THE PSYCHOLOGIST

Clinical psychologists work in a wide range of situations: with elderly people, mentally handicapped adults and children, violent offenders, families, chronic pain patients and various other disorders and groups. The psychologist's role involves detailed assessment of the person, the attendant circumstances and the social context within which the 'problem' is occurring. The assessment may involve the use of a variety of psychological tests and the interpretation of them (Roth, 1990).

Clinical psychologists are subject to the codes of practice of the British Psychological Society, and they operate within the guidelines of their employer. The problems referred to clinical psychologists may have several causes. The psychologist is involved in the assessment of a problem in relation to the origin, whether it is psychological or physical in origin. However the problem may have both elements, closely inter-related.

Social context

Behaviour cannot be labelled as a problem without considering the social context in which it occurs. For example, a woman who talks to people who are not physically present and who reports hearing voices might be judged to have a problem. If certain other symptoms are present, she might be described as psychotic. However, if she claims to be a medium and assists people in getting in touch with their dead relatives, then her behaviour might be regarded as socially acceptable.

Rosenhan (1973) carried out a study on the effects of social labelling. In this study eight subjects were instructed to claim that they had heard voices in order to gain admission to mental institutions. They were labelled as schizophrenics. Once in the institutions they behaved normally, claiming that they now felt better and the symptoms had disappeared. The other patients accepted that they were normal but the staff continued to believe they were insane and they were only released when the hospital was told about the experiment. The staff saw the diary-keeping of one subject as a further symptom of his problem. Another subject was labelled as showing signs of social withdrawal because he did not wish to join in social activities and other subjects, who tried to convince staff of their true identity, were seen as having delusions.

Clinical psychologists carry out evaluation and research in the areas in which they work and may also evaluate the effectiveness of a particular type of service. They also work in multidisciplinary teams, which leads to a sharing of knowledge and methods of enquiry and assessment. Psychologists need to be aware of biological factors and how they interact with external experiences. They often use behaviour modification or the cognitive behavioural approach in treatment.

Assessment of pain

Psychological factors play an important role in pain perception and evidence relating to suggestion and placebo medication supports the view that psychological processes operating to produce pain relief can help a number of sufferers. Reliable and valid assessment is necessary for any evaluation of therapeutic outcome. Assessing pain is not easy since it is a subjective phenomenon. Various methods have been developed that impose structure on the assessment of pain perception. Two most frequently used are the visual analogue scales and the McGill Pain Questionnaire (MPQ) (see Chapter 5). Other assessments used may measure pain locus of control, positive and negative affect, beliefs and attitudes, and anxiety and depression.

The psychological approach to pain management

The most popular methods are distraction and relaxation and biofeedback. All these techniques have been shown to work with acute pain but on their own are ultimately ineffective with chronic pain over a long period. The most effective approach for chronic pain has been shown to be the cognitive behavioural approach, combined with the group concept. The work carried out by Fordyce (1982) supports this. Psychologists are usually instrumental in setting this up and acting as team leaders for the multidisciplinary team.

THE PAIN TEAM

The multidisciplinary team approach has been shown to benefit the patient (Mayer *et al.*, 1987; Murphy, 1987; Hazard *et al.*, 1989). Research has shown that the utilization of several treatment approaches in chronic pain relief gives a higher success rate than when just one approach is used. The group approach provides a mutual support network for the patients and a forum within which they have shared experiences, symptoms and fears. The aims of chronic pain groups are that the participants will learn to manage their pain, have confidence in their own abilities and become less reliant on the medical profession.

The team approach is an extension of the unidisciplinary model where we have the doctor–patient or therapist–patient interaction. Team members usually belong to one or more of the following disciplines: physiotherapy, occupational therapy, clinical psychology and nursing. The philosophies and core skills provided by the team members are complementary to each other and to the interventions offered by the pain consultant. Therapists provide treatment programmes which are given in parallel or sequentially within the outpatient, inpatient or domiciliary setting. The aim of this intervention is educative and participative, encouraging the patient to play an active part.

Parallel therapy model

If the team is working within the parallel therapy model (Figure 10.1) it maximizes the benefit that can be obtained from a single treatment option.

For example, the physiotherapist may mobilize a limb following a guanethidine block so that active and passive movement are facilitated while the limb is pain-free. The patient will then have treatment from the occupational therapist and physiotherapist as part of their ongoing treatment programme. Using a combination of nerve block, manipulation, occupational therapy and physiotherapy is a common procedure in the treatment of reflex sympathetic dystrophy (Hardy and Hill, 1990).

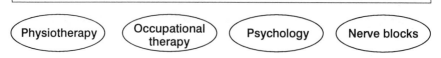

Figure 10.1   Parallel therapy model.

Sequential therapy model

In the sequential therapy model (Figure 10.2) several techniques are used for pain management.

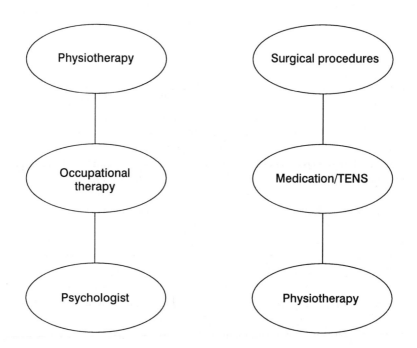

Figure 10.2   Sequential therapy model.

Each treatment is offered for a set period of time and the patient undergoes each phase of the treatment in turn. For example they may be treated by medication, then referred to physiotherapy and then have a course of occupational therapy. In some pain programmes this model is used with each treatment modality lasting for 2 months. 'In one phase an injection (epidural or facet joint block) is given with physiotherapy; in a second phase a transcutaneous electrical nerve stimulator is demonstrated and used; and in a third phase treatments based on psychological theory are taught and used' (Hardy and Hill, 1990) The patient is assessed before and during the programme using the doctor–patient interaction format. The sequential therapy model of treatment can be adapted for use with chronic pelvic pain and facial pain.

Interdisciplinary team approach

'Interdisciplinary' is now considered to be a more accurate title for teams working with groups within the pain clinic environment. 'Multidisciplinary' is used for teams within wards where several disciplines work together in a specific directorate, such as orthopaedics, but each deliver their treatment individually, either in the parallel or sequential model. The interdisciplinary team members have a unified approach, philosophy and goals and the emphasis is on a single coordinated result. The aim is not cure but self-management through the use of learned coping skills and education in pain management. The team members all adopt a consistent approach and although there may be an overlap in their roles they are also complementary. The patient is not passed from department to department for treatment but has the benefit of an interdisciplinary approach during the treatment. All members of the team are fully conversant with the other members' roles and are able to take on these roles if necessary. For example, both the psychologist and occupational therapist may carry out the teaching of relaxation techniques and the physiotherapist, psychologist and occupational therapist will all contribute to the teaching of goal-setting and pacing (Figure 10.3). Although there is a consequent blurring of individual roles this approach is more effective than the sequential or parallel therapy model. Individual team members retain their professional identity but present a unified approach with shared treatment goals.

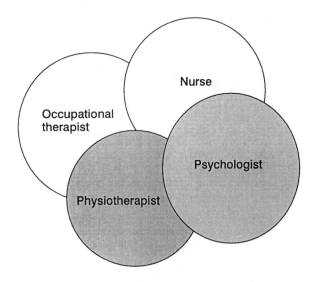

Figure 10.3 Interdisciplinary role overlap.

Types of programme

There are different levels of programmes within this approach. The first-level programme is educative. Patients attend short courses consisting of four weekly sessions. They are taught simple techniques aimed at maintaining an optimum level of activity and function. Education is received about their medical condition and general functioning of the body in relation to posture. Patients are usually in full-time work and this type of programme has a preventative bias. It is suitable for back education, irritable bowel syndrome and stress management.

The second-level programme is educative, with a more detailed programme relating to stress management, problem-solving and task management. It has a stronger rehabilitative bias. This type of programme may run for 6 weeks with one session per week. The patients usually have problems that are not chronic but are no longer in the acute phase. Groups may consist of patients with multi-pain problems such as abdominal, facial, neck and shoulder pains. Special groups may be run for patients with a single diagnosis, such as back pain.

The third type of programme is at the chronic pain level. It is more intensive and patients attend between two and five days per week for a period of 4–6 weeks. This type may be run as an inpatient programme or as a combination of inpatient and outpatient. In the latter case the patients attend as inpatients for 1–2 weeks and then one day a week for several weeks as outpatients. They have a further week as inpatients towards the end of the course. Some programmes are also run on an overlap principle. Group 1 will be halfway through their programme when group 2 starts; this has the advantage that the second group are encouraged by the first group's progress. The first group of patients is also able to offer advice and support to the new group. In chronic pain management this format is usually used with inpatient programmes. The inpatient programme is more intensive and addresses the problems of drug dependency more specifically, as well as the areas indicated in the other programmes.

Taylor *et al.* (1980) found that patients who are treated in this way could increase their activity time by up to 91% at discharge. They used fewer medical resources and the improved quality of life, mood and physical ability was measurable.

Many studies have shown significant increases in activity levels, which are maintained up to 3 years after treatment. Pinsky (1983) found that following treatment medication was reduced, as was use of health-care facilities. Painter, Seres and Newman (1980) found that up to 61% of patients may not require any medical assistance for up to 2 years after discharge. Even domiciliary programmes have shown a 70% change in lifestyle (Corey, Etlin and Miller, 1987). In a study carried out by Richardson *et al.* (1994) on quality of work and employment status of chronic pain patients on a pain management programme, the findings suggest that this approach benefits both the unemployed and those in employment. The work performance of employed patients improved and the likelihood of employment for those unemployed increased. Those patients who had returned to work, even for a short period of time, showed an improvement at 1-year follow-up in pain measures, self-confidence and the effect of pain on daily living. Richardson *et al.* state that this improvement is possibly due to 'the beneficial effects of return to work on patients' psychological adjustment rather than *vice versa*'. Return to work is dependent on several variables, such as the requirements of the job, the flexibility of the workplace and the current job market and economic climate.

Advantages of the interdisciplinary approach

The interdisciplinary team is a group of different professional people working together to provide a direct client-care service. All team members are aware of the role and function of the team and are working to achieve the same goals. Each member of the team has his/her role; often these will merge, resulting in a blurring of roles. This can be an advantage, as patients do not have to rely on one particular person or discipline for advice in any one area. Team members act as facilitators, enabling clients to take control of their lives and live as normal a life as possible. The support of the team for each other means that no member of the team works in isolation. Each member of the team has their own personal skills and experience; as these are all different this enhances and enlarges the skills and experience of the team as a unit (Table 10.1).

Table 10.1 Advantages and disadvantages of interdisciplinary approach

Advantages	Disadvantages
Patients do not become dependent on one member of staff	Some patients feel intimidated by the group approach
Team members do not work in isolation	Team members come from differing professional backgrounds
Individual skills and experience enhance the abilities of the team as a whole	If there is no team leader the team may lack cohesiveness
Interdisciplinary team meetings	Poor interteam communication
Team members provide support for each other	Blurring of roles may cause professional rivalry

Disadvantages of the interdisciplinary approach

This approach is not ideal for all patients, as some will feel intimidated by the group situation and would be better dealt with on an individual basis. It is essential for each team member to be committed to the overall philosophy for it to be effective. This is sometimes difficult as each discipline's immediate supervisor is not a member of the team. However this is tending to alter as teams move into clinical directorates where they are seen as one entity, not a collection of different professionals.

To function effectively there needs to be one team member who is designated either 'director' or 'team leader'. In the majority of teams this role is taken by the psychologist. If there is no 'leader' the team may not be cohesive and members may work in parallel, instead of together and with each other, causing alienation of individual team members. Although there should be agreement on the philosophy of the team it is important that each team member maintains their professional identity. If they are not sure of their professional role this can lead to ineffectiveness and loss of respect for the others' professions. This, along with professional rivalry, can be detrimental to the patient's needs. Good communication is essential; the holding of weekly meetings to discuss philosophy and strategies will ensure that good communication is maintained

PRACTICAL ADVICE FOR SETTING UP A PAIN MANAGEMENT PROGRAMME

Pain clinics were set up in the United Kingdom in the 1960s. John Lloyd and Sam Lipton, two anaesthetists with an interest in pain, were at the forefront of this innovation. They recognized the need for a service for patients suffering from pain. The techniques used at that time were nerve blocks and pharmacological interventions. Today the interventions have extended to include the management of both physical and psychological aspects of acute and chronic pain. The interventions offered now include group sessions that have an interdisciplinary approach. Many pain clinics now offer pain management programmes as well as the traditional interventions. Ideally the pain clinic will have an anaesthetist, specialist nurse, physiotherapist, occupational therapist and psychologist in the core team, with other disciplines such as social worker, dietician and acupuncturist being involved when necessary.

In 1993 a working party carried out a survey of the facilities provided by pain clinics. Their findings indicate that patients who are treated on pain management programmes use far fewer health-care resources following discharge. The working party also suggested that interdisciplinary pain management is a more accurate description of current methodology in the UK (Working Party, 1993). The interdisciplinary approach, where the assessment process is coordinated by the pain management service and treatment is based on the assessment outcome, has been found to be more cost-effective than the multidisciplinary approach.

Pain management programmes

This approach is widely used in pain management both on an individual and group treatment basis. Behavioural programmes for chronic pain patients have been running in America for many years since the pioneering work of Wilbert Fordyce and work by Dennis Turk, who incorporated cognitive-behavioural techniques into chronic pain management. This approach does not depend on the identification of a treatable cause for the pain but looks at the level of dysfunction and stress caused by it. The behavioural adaptations used in acute pain, such as resting, time off work, help from others, tend to become permanent features of the individual's coping strategy in chronic pain. Patients become depressed and anxious when the pain fails to respond to treatment or behavioural modification. Behavioural adaptations and modifications that are used to cope with the pain become established habits or behaviours in the life of the individual.

The aims of the cognitive behavioural approach are to improve coping skills and general fitness levels, to reduce stress and tension and to enable the patient to have control of the pain. This is achieved by the maintenance of an operant environment where change can be affected in activities, behaviour, thoughts and feelings. This can occur even if there is no change in pain intensity.

Operant environment

All staff involved in the pain management programme should be familiar with the concepts of operant conditioning. The staff reinforce all well behaviours and ignore any pain or illness behaviour. It is easier to maintain this if the pain management centre is outside the hospital and the staff are not in uniform. To facilitate a change in habits and behaviour patients are taught about the 'model of chronic pain'. This is a two-way communication process utilizing the group's experience. Members of the group are encouraged to identify areas of change, any problems that might be encountered and any factors that might be helpful in accomplishing change. The cognitive techniques used in chronic pain management are based on methods used in the treatment of anxiety and depression. Patients are taught to recognize the fact that anxiety levels rise when the pain increases and to accept that they may fail because they have set too high a goal. Beliefs about pain that are reinforcing the invalid status are challenged. The patients are encouraged to set more realistic goals, to appreciate their strengths and to be less critical of their performance.

Operant conditioning applied to the pain programme

Patients on a pain management course are taught to pace their exercises and each individual decides on the level and amount of exercise they are able to do. They then learn how to adapt the pacing concept to any activity they undertake. Patients are also taught how to set base lines for activity. They learn about their body, how it functions and why inactivity can increase the pain.

Patients are taught goal-setting and are shown how to set long-term and short-term goals that are realistic, achievable, specific and relevant. Body mechanics are taught on the course, so that unnecessary pain and strain can be avoided when carrying out activities. Communication issues are covered, as changing one's behaviour can affect family and friends.

Research has shown that opiates, antidepressants and tranquillizers are often ineffective and can cause side effects such as drowsiness, dry mouth, constipation, memory problems and lack of concentration. The advantages and disadvantages of taking medication are discussed with the patient and medication is reduced with guidance in gradual stages. Many patients have difficulty sleeping, which affects their mood and activity levels during the day. Patients are taught how to improve their sleep pattern so that they are more in control.

Patients are taught relaxation skills to enable them to cope with the pain. Simple techniques are used which focus on breathing and the overall reduction of muscle tension. Other techniques use mental imagery, distraction and focusing techniques.

To enable patients to understand their chronic pain problem information and discussion about current theories of pain and the rationale behind various treatments is used. This also gives the patients an opportunity to express some of their frustration and disappointment with previous treatment and to adjust their expectations of treatment to a more realistic level.

A suggested outline programme for pain management is given in Table 10.2.

Guidelines for chronic pain management

At present there are no official guidelines for pain management for chronic pain patients or a relevant programme. The suggestions in Table 10.3 are based on the author's own experience in the chronic pain field and the proposed definitions/descriptions/criteria for pain management programmes currently being formulated by the Pain Society.

Selection of patients

The selection of patients usually depends on the referrals from other health-care professionals. However, many therapists and nurses are now involved in the assessment process prior to the patient being offered a place on a pain programme. Patients must be able to commit themselves to regular attendance for the duration of the course. They also have to be prepared to arrange transport as there is usually no transport entitlement for this kind of treatment. Staff should have access to information on the local 'dial a ride' service and other local voluntary transport schemes. Group programmes may not be appropriate for patients who have psychiatric problems or a psychological problem such as unresolved bereavement. Other contraindications are high levels of dependence on family members and inflexible psychosocial networks relating to the individual's problems. All patients must have had the relevant investigations to eliminate any underlying pathological cause.

Table 10.2 Outline programme for pain management

Week	Pain model	Information	Exercise	Relaxation	Practical
1	Three systems model	Aims of group Seating	Introduction to exercise	Introduction to stress and relaxation	Breathing exercise Exercises
2	Activities Goal-setting	Pacing		Deep muscle relaxation	Exercises Relaxation
3	Pain pathways Gate control theory	Lifting TENS			Exercises Relaxation
4	Thoughts and feelings	Drugs and doctors	Benefits of exercise and fitness	Self-hypnosis	Exercises Relaxation
5	Pain behaviours and communication	Activities of daily living	Exercise fitness circuit	Autogenic relaxation	Exercises Relaxation
6	Sleep	Beds and sleeping	Exercise circuit	Application of relaxation	Exercises Relaxation

Table 10.3   Summary of guidelines for a chronic pain programme

Selection of patients Selection criteria	Referral from medical and other health-care professionals Patient must be able to attend regularly Patients should not be undergoing any other pain treatment Patients should not have psychiatric problems Patients must want to change their lifestyle
Resources required	Suitable group room Secretarial and photocopying facilities Time for report writing and team meetings
Format of programme	Number of sessions per week Number of weeks course will run Inpatient or outpatient Follow-up sessions
Staffing levels – core team	Pain consultant Psychologist Physiotherapist Nurse Occupational therapist
Other team members	Secretarial assistance Acupuncturist Dietician Pharmacist

Staffing levels

Ideally, a core team for pain management groups should include a nurse, phys-iotherapist, occupational therapist, psychologist and medical doctor (with pain as a specialist area), plus secretarial assistance. However, there are pain management programmes which are run, due to difficulties recruiting, with only three core team members. 'Staff should be educated and trained in the models and skills required and have research based knowledge of the area in which they work. Visits to existing pain management programmes can facilitate guidance and access to pain management literature, and provide observation of the skills required, but these do not constitute training. Training may also be available, but is not yet formalized' (Seers *et al.*, 1994)

Resources required for the programme

'The programme should have a designated space for its activities' (International Association for the Study of Pain, 1990). The allocated room should be large enough for a group of patients to use exercise mats and to lie down for relax-ation. Group sizes vary around the country from 8–14. There should be easy access to toilets and tea-making facilities. Ideally, secretarial facilities and office space should be adjacent to the group room but in many cases this is situated elsewhere. The hours allocated to team members should include time for team meetings, paperwork and training. 'Staff should teach other health care professionals and promote awareness in the lay public' (International Association for the Study of Pain, 1990).

Format of the programme

When setting up a programme the following issues need to be addressed. How many sessions per week? How long is a session? How many weeks will the course run for? Often this depends on the availability of resources. Outpatient programmes usually run two sessions per week for 6 weeks. Sessions will last from 2.5–3 hours. Usually, patients are reassessed at 6 weeks post-group and 6 months post-group, so that the course can be evaluated. Several programmes also have a 3-month follow-up session. There are currently several inpatient programmes running in England and Wales, which include Input, St Thomas' Hospital, London, the Royal National Hospital for Rheumatic Disease in Bath, Unsted Park Rehabilitation Hospital in Surrey and the Input Pain Management Centre, Bronllys Hospital in Brecon.

Guidelines for acute pain

Clinical guidelines for the management of acute pain are due to be published in 1996 by the NHS Executive Nursing Directorate. These guidelines have a multidisciplinary input and the key principles will cover the management of acute pain in adults, in the hospital and community.

The general principles which underpin all sections of this document are that pain management is an integral part of effective health care. Pain management is individual to each patient and prevention of pain should be a primary aim of all health-care professionals. It is a multiprofessional activity that acknowledges the important role of the patient and the facilitating of the two-way exchange of information between patient and professional. When managing acute pain, culture, pain perception and attitudes of both patients and staff play an important part in treatment. Although pain is complex and subjective it has quantifiable features, which include time-course, intensity, individual perception and the effect on the individual. The draft guidelines recommend that there should be continuity of management in relation to medication and other management techniques when the patient moves from the hospital to the community, and *vice versa*. Staff should have good communication skills and adequate education and training. It is also recommended that patients should have written information on pain management options available to them so that they are able to make an informed choice.

The document contains key principles for acute pain assessment, pharmacological management of acute pain, non-pharmacological management of acute pain, evaluation of effectiveness, education and training and a reference section and a literature review.

11 | Pain-allied disorders

BACK PAIN

Back pain and injury constitute an ongoing and increasing problem and there are many causes of back pain. Common causes are disc herniation and arthritis of the vertebral joints. However, 60–78% of patients with low back pain have no apparent physical signs of injury (Loeser, 1980). In acute episodes of back pain the onset is sudden and often resolves with rest and medication followed by a gradual increase of activity and exercise. Back pain can become a chronic or frequently recurring problem resulting in a change of work status, lifestyle and restriction of social activities. Chronic back pain is often accompanied by anxiety, depression and stress-related disorders.

Prolapsed or herniated intervertebral disc

This is often referred to as a 'slipped disc'. The disc does not slip out of position, as the common term suggests, but is usually torn and there is a leakage of the central soft area of the disc. It is this mechanical pressure of the prolapsed disc on the nerve root that causes local inflammation, which in turn causes pain. Only 60% of patients with disc herniation and associated sciatic pain have relief from surgery. Discectomy has most effect in those patients who have clear evidence of nerve root compression. Disc herniation is often the result of a bending or twisting action, e.g. pushing the car, pulling up weeds in the garden or moving awkward or heavy objects. It can also be the result of repetitive strain on the back through bad working posture and environment or prolonged sitting or bending postures required to carry out the job. Examples of this are computer operators, jobs that involve long-distance car driving on a regular basis and jobs with a high stress element. In the current job climate many people are unable to pace their activities as they are constrained by deadlines and increased work loads.

Degenerative or wear-and-tear changes

Disc spaces may become narrow as the discs lose some of their fluid and there-fore some of their shock-absorbing qualities. Spinal joints may wear and inflammation, pain and stiffness are a common symptom of this. Bony spikes (osteophytes) may develop and in time the foramen are narrowed, causing stenosis. As the foramen narrows, blood circulation to the nerves can also be affected, resulting in pins and needles, numbness or pain in the legs on walking. Stenosis may cause irritation of the nerve root, resulting in inflammation, pain and stiffness. Sometimes a decompression operation is carried out to widen the foramen and release pressure on the nerves. Disorders such as ankylosing spondylitis, rheumatoid arthritis and arachnoiditis may cause localized inflam-mation, pain and discomfort and are usually treated with medication, rest and sometimes injections until the symptoms subside.

Surgery

In reality only a few back-pain complaints are helped by surgery. Operations tend to cause inflammation in the same way as trauma. Successive back surgery is rarely successful and often causes more inflammation, scarring and pain than the original procedure.

Strains and sprains

The ligaments and muscles that surround the spine can be sprained or strained in exactly the same way as other joints in the body, which can lead to pain. Poor posture due to bad working positions, poor seating or slouching and being over-weight can put strain on joints, muscles and ligaments. This type of back pain usually responds to rest, physiotherapy and advice on care of the back.

Backache is quite a common symptom, like a headache. Occasionally it can become acutely painful, sometimes because of accident but often there is no attributable cause. Unaccustomed work entailing bending or spells of work which is heavier than usual are contributory factors to the onset of back pain. Loeser (1980) and Watts (1985) found that over 50% of people following episodes of low back pain were symptom-free within 2 months with no health-care intervention.

Initially rest is recommended in the acute phase followed by a graded exer-cise regime and education in care of the back. In more chronic cases relaxation and stress management, behaviour modification and a change in lifestyle can be beneficial. Other techniques and procedures which may be used are TENS, acupuncture, nerve blocks and pharmaceutical interventions. Swanson *et al.* (1976) found that the most effective form of treatment for back pain was one that used a combination of various techniques and therapies.

CANCER PAIN

Cancer is rarely painful during the early stages as most tumours grow very slowly. Twycross and Lack (1990) estimate that two-thirds of patients with cancer experience pain. Pain may not be apparent until the diagnostic or therapy stage of the cancer and in some cases it is only present in the later stages of the disease. Pain is usually caused when the tumour starts to impede or occlude various structures. Patients with metastatic cancer usually develop pain which increases in severity. Brain tumours may cause severe headaches and abdominal cancers may cause obstruction in the intestine, bladder, ureter or bile ducts. Bone tumours may weaken the periosteum, causing pathological fractures. If the bony tumour is in the bones of the vertebral column the consequent collapse of the vertebrae causes damage to the sensory nerve roots. Pain may also be caused by muscle spasm, lymphoedema and myopathy. Treatment may cause pain, e.g. following operation, postoperative complications and post radiation fibrosis. The cancer and its treatment may cause associated pain through constipation, post-hepetic neuralgia and decubitus ulcer. Patients may also suffer from pain unrelated to the cancer, such as musculoskeletal pain and migraines.

The term 'total pain' in relation to terminal illness as cited by Dame Cicely Saunders (1989) is often used. 'The concept is based on observations that an individual's experience of pain is a combination of emotional, spiritual and social pain as well as physical pain' (Pearce, 1995). The change of role within the family, or loss of role, perception of body image, inability to carry out leisure or social activities, and the fear of dying, contribute to the complexity of the situation, often resulting in feelings of anger, frustration and depression. The cancer patient often feels that they have lost control not only physically but emotionally as well.

Treatments which may be used include surgery, chemotherapy and radiotherapy. Medication may include tricyclic antidepressants for the dull aching neuropathic pain but these may be of limited benefit. Relaxation, stress management, pacing, energy conservation and counselling are also used in the treatment of cancer pain. Any therapy offered is curative or, in the advanced stages, aimed at symptom control or relief. Patient education should relate to the illness, its treatment, self-help techniques and support mechanisms available for the patient and their relatives.

HEAD AND FACE PAIN SYNDROMES

Trigeminal neuralgia (also called tic douloureux) and migraines are two of the commonest pain syndromes seen in the head and face. Pain in the head or face is also associated with brain tumours.

Trigeminal neuralgia

This pain syndrome is a disorder of sensory fibres of the trigeminal (fifth cranial) nerve. It is seen more often in older people and is characterized by recurrent episodes of excruciating pain along the nerve pathways. The pain is often described as stabbing in nature and lasts for seconds to minutes. Onset may be spontaneous but can also be precipitated by light touch or facial movement, e.g. washing the face, eating. When the pain is recurrent it is often accompanied by depression. The cause of the neuralgia is unknown. Stress management, relaxation, nerve blocks and drug therapy may be used in the treatment of this disorder. When drug therapy is unsuccessful peripheral nerve blocks are carried out. Peripheral nerve blocks using glycerol are effective for long periods and do not impair facial sensation. Freezing of the nerve (cryoanalgesia) under local anaesthetic can also be used.

Migraines

A total of 20% of the population suffer from migraine and although there is no evidence that anxiety and tension are the cause of the condition they can exacerbate it. Usually the onset of a migraine is accompanied by visual disturbances. These take the form of bright spots, jagged streaks of light and even loss of vision in one eye. One of the main features of migraines is that they are unilateral. In severe cases this is accompanied by pins and needles or numbness of the hands or face. Transient weakness of a limb, or in some cases half of the body, may also occur. Symptoms usually subside after 15–30 minutes and the sufferer then experiences severe pain on one side of the head, which may persist for several days. At its peak the headache may be accompanied by nausea and vomiting.

The above signs and symptoms relate to 'classical migraine'. In 'atypical migraine' the headache occurs in the absence of other symptoms and may be accompanied by vomiting; this is the commonest form of migraine. There is a higher prevalence in women and it is most common between 20 and 40 years of age.

These disorders are often treated with medication and the teaching of stress and relaxation techniques.

OSTEOARTHRITIS

Osteoarthritis is a degenerative disease of the joints usually accompanied by pain and stiffness. Although it has a higher incidence in women over the age of 55 this disorder affects both sexes. The most frequent sites of degeneration are the weight-bearing joints such as hips and knees and the interphalangeal joints of the fingers. In the advanced stages of the disease pain is also present at rest.

As joints become stiffer and more painful there is a loss of mobility and muscle wasting can occur. Although 80% of people between the ages of 55 and 64 will show changes characteristic of osteoarthritis on X-ray, only 20% complain of symptoms. Occupation, trauma, sport and obesity are considered to be contributory factors in the development of this disease.

Osteoarthritis is treated by drug therapy, physiotherapy, occupational therapy and surgical intervention such as hip and knee replacements. Although drug therapy can help in this condition the side effects of NSAIDs preclude their long-term use. Pre- and postoperatively the patient may need aids and adaptations to the home and advice from the occupational therapist and physiotherapist on exercise, pacing of activity and relaxation.

PHANTOM LIMB PAIN

Hodges and Bender (1994) estimate that 60–80% of people experience phantom limb pain following amputation. Phantom limb pain also occurs in brachial plexus avulsions and spinal cord injuries.

The majority of amputees experience occasional episodes of pain and many have clinically significant phantom limb pain. This is thought to be physiological in origin and is due to the decreased blood flow and microspasms in the residual limb. This causes referred pain into the phantom limb. Other causes are thought to be due to the prosthesis; this results in a burning, cramping phantom pain. In postamputation syndrome the pain may be localized to the stump, there may be pain in the phantom limb and sensations may be experienced in the phantom limb. Sherman (1994) states that 'treatments related to specific symptomology can be effective'. Treatments include peripheral vasodilators, muscle relaxants and biofeedback but no effective treatment has been found for shooting pain. Although sympathectomy can be successful in the treatment of burning pain, the pain may recur or increase after a year. Prolonged standing and physical activity tend to exacerbate the pain.

Phantom phenomenon following spinal cord injury occurs after several months and the patient is only able to give a vague description of the limb. In postamputation syndrome the phantom limb can telescope into the stump; this does not occur in spinal cord injury (Wall, 1981)

Other techniques and treatments which may help the patient to cope with the pain are relaxation and stress management, pacing of activity, TENS, ultrasound, nerve blocks and medication.

REFLEX SYMPATHETIC DYSTROPHY

Reflex sympathetic dystrophy (RSD) is defined by the International Association for the Study of Pain as 'continuous pain in a portion of an extremity after trauma which may include fracture but does not involve a major nerve, associated with sympathetic hyperactivity'.

This disorder is known by many different names, e.g. Sudeck's atrophy, osteodystrophy, disuse atrophy and a variety of other synonyms (Table 11.1).

Table 11.1 Reflex sympathetic dystrophy: some terms used for this condition and some of the predisposing conditions

Terms used	Predisposing conditions
Algoneurodystrophy	Blunt trauma (often trivial)
Chronic traumatic oedema	Burns
Minor or major causalgia	Cerebal infarction
Post-traumatic pain syndrome	Cervical spondylosis
Reflex algodystrophy	Gunshot wound
Reflex sympathetic dystrophy	Surgery
Sudeck's atrophy	Myocardial infarction
Shoulder–hand syndrome	Inflammatory disorders
Sympathalgia	Degenerative joint disease

The name many occupational therapists know it by is **Sudeck's atrophy**. Paul Hermann Sudeck was a German surgeon who described a type of acute bone atrophy in 1900. However, this reference was to acute inflammatory bone atrophy rather than to post-traumatic atrophy following fracture.

The earliest descriptions of the syndrome are by Mitchell, Morehouse and Keen (1864) during the American Civil War; they observed that soldiers with high-velocity missile wounds had persistent pain accompanied by vasomotor changes and they labelled this condition **causalgia** (*caus* = 'burning'; *algia* = 'pain') The term **reflex sympathetic dystrophy** was introduced by Evans in 1947 (Patt and Balter, 1991) and is used in a generic way to a range of post-traumatic soft tissue injuries accompanied by vasomotor changes. More recently, 'sympathetically maintained', or 'sympathetic-dependent' has been suggested as a more appropriate description (Churcher and Ingall, 1987).

Reflex sympathetic dystrophy most commonly follows minor trauma injuries such as sprain, Colles fracture and Dupuytren's contracture. Less frequently it follows crush injuries and peripheral nerve involvement. It is difficult to quantify the actual incidence of this diagnosis as many are not diagnosed until they have had the symptoms for some time. The patient may have suffered pain or dysfunction for over 12 months. The severity of the injury bears little or no relation to the incidence of the condition.

The affected limb presents as painful and swollen. It may change colour and is hypersensitive to touch. There may also be temperature changes to the affected limb. Other characteristics are marked joint stiffness and signs of osteoporosis on X-ray.

There are generally three stages of RSD (Table 11.2).

Table 11.2 Symptoms and stages of reflex sympathetic dystrophy

Symptoms	Stage 1 0–3 months	Stage 2 3–12 months	Stage 3 months to years
Pain	Burning increasing	Gets worse if untreated Aggravated by movement	Reaches peak? Improves slowly
Swelling	Soft pitting oedema	Hard oedema Elevation little effect	Periarticular thickening of joints
Stiffness	Progressive	Progressive	If persists, may lead to deformities
Discoloration	Pale/red/blotchy	Redness	Pale
Osteoporosis	Present at 3–5 weeks	Demineralization increases	Widespread
Sudomotor	Sweaty ++	Less sweating	Dry
Temperature	Coolness	Increased heat	Cool
Vasomotor	Vasoconstriction	Vasolability	Vasoconstriction
Trophic		Atrophy of skin and subcutaneous tissue	Glossy appearance
Fibrotic		Palmar fascitis nodules Thickening of longitudinal bands	As stage 2 ++

The initial stage (acute) has a duration of 3 months and may subside spontaneously or respond rapidly to treatment. Pain, swelling, vasodilatation and joint stiffness are the main characteristics.

Stage 2 (subacute) may last from 3–6 months. At this stage pain increases and becomes more diffuse, oedema spreads and becomes hard rather than soft, nails become brittle, cracked or grooved. Spotty osteoporosis occurs early but may become severe and diffuse at this stage. There is a thickening of joints and muscle wasting.

By stage 3 (chronic) the limb shows marked trophic changes, which eventually become irreversible, pain may become intractable and involve the entire limb, muscles atrophy and joints become weak and may finally become ankylosed. Contractures of the flexor tendons may occur and bone deossification is marked and diffuse.

Primary causes are often defined as surgery, trauma, infections, cerebral lesions, spinal and spinal cord dysfunction, and ischaemic heart disease (Table 11.3).

Table 11.3 Disorders referred to as reflex sympathetic dystrophy and causes

Minor causalgia	Involvement of peripheral nerve
Minor traumatic dystrophy	Commonest type
	Initial injury may be fracture, dislocation
	Degree of involvement may only be single digit
Shoulder–hand syndrome	Caused by proximal trauma such as shoulder neck or rib cage injury
	Starts with pain and stiffness in shoulder radiating to whole limb
Major traumatic dystrophy	Follows Colles fracture, crush injury
	Presents with pain, stiffness, swelling
Major causalgia	Injury to major mixed nerve in the proximal part of the extremity

Cailliet (1992) considers that the most frequent cause in the lower limb is following surgical intervention, the application of tight casts and injuries near to or of the lower limb nerves. However one third or more of RSD patients have no definitive precipitating factors.

Treatment of this condition is most successful at stages one and two. A combination of therapies such as nerve blocks, physiotherapy and occupational therapy is effective in the treatment of this disorder. Specific techniques or modalities used may include tricyclic drugs (such as amitriptyline), sympathetic nerve blocks, TENS, graded exercise and activity programme within the limits of the pain and desensitization. Pacing of activities and the use of resting splints are also useful.

REPETITIVE STRAIN INJURY

Repetitive strain injury (RSI) is a general term for musculoskeletal disorders that involve all or part of the upper limbs, including the neck. This group of disorders is often referred to as work-related upper limb disorders (WRULDS). Disorders that come into this category are carpal tunnel syndrome, compression neuropathy, de Quervain's disease, tendinitis, tenosynovitis, bursitis, lateral epicondylitis and medial epicondylitis. The symptoms may include pain, discomfort, aching, paraesthesia, anaesthesia, weakness, tenderness, burning, swelling and restriction of movement. Often the symptoms are poorly localized and non-specific. Disorders of the soft tissues, tendons, nerves and muscles are frequently seen in the upper limb as a result of repetitive movements and overexertion.

RSI is a muscle overuse syndrome (Pearson, 1990) and is a result of excessive or incorrect use of the limb. We now know that there are causal links between specific occupations and hand/wrist disorders. In the ergonomic and biomechanics fields there is also evidence relating to job demands that incorporate physical stresses.

Factors that play a part are the amount of force applied, the frequency and duration of movement, or the repetition element and the posture involved. RSI is seen in many occupations, including musicians, computer operators, factory workers, housewives with small children and students. In the last the condition is often triggered by concentrated hours of writing during exams. RSI is a progressive condition but it may be triggered by a single traumatic event.

The condition can be managed with rest, medication, adaptation of the environment, the use of ergonomic principles and pacing of activity. Treatment may also include ultrasound, icing or contrast baths, anti-inflammatory drugs, exercise, relaxation and stress management, education in relation to the management and cause of the condition.

RHEUMATOID ARTHRITIS

Rheumatoid arthritis is a chronic systemic disease of unknown aetiology. It is seen more often in women than men and the average age of onset is between 25 and 55. The condition has an insidious onset and initially the symptoms are those of general fatigue and non-specific illness, with stiffness and tenderness in the joints. The hands, feet, wrists, elbows and knees are usually the first to be affected. The progress of the disease is symmetrical and the joints become red, swollen and painful making movement difficult. If early treatment is not available there is progressive destruction of the joints and the development of deformity leading to permanent disability. Rheumatoid arthritis is a systemic disease which affects all aspects of daily life. Treatment may include medication, splinting to prevent deformity of joints, physiotherapy, occupational therapy and in some cases surgery.

SHOULDER–HAND SYNDROME

This may follow a frozen shoulder, stroke or trauma to the shoulder. It is sometimes referred to as causalgia or reflex dystrophy (see above). Symptoms are pain in the shoulder, oedema, pain and vasomotor changes in the hand (Cailliet, 1991). The patient experiences pain and has a restricted range of movement and a dysfunctional hand. Treatment includes reduction of oedema through elevation, a paced exercise and therapy regime within the limits of the pain and relaxation. Frozen shoulders are usually treated by the administration of a steroid injection followed by physiotherapy.

THALAMIC PAIN

Thalamic pain occurs in 2% of stroke patients. It can develop immediately post-stroke or may occur many months later. It does not respond to analgesics or narcotics and surgical intervention has minimal success. Tricyclic antidepressants tend to have a positive response and are used in a low dosage. TENS has a variable response.

Noback and Demarest (1977) stated that thalamic lesions may produce 'thalamic syndrome'. This may result in loss or impaired sensation contralaterally, or overactive sensory responses with pain and discomfort. Levenson (1971) and Guyton (1981) also considered that occlusion to the thalamus may result in loss of contralateral sensation and the patient may experience unpleasant distortions of cutaneous sensation with burning pain which occurs spontaneously. Patients describe the pain as burning, shooting and throbbing. The pain may affect the whole side of the body affected by the stroke or only a small part. Sensation is always abnormal in the affected area and there is a decrease in pinprick sensation and awareness of temperature. The pain is activated by cutaneous stimulation and temperature changes. Many patients find that rubbing the affected limb can precipitate it. Thalamic pain is seen more often in the under-60 age group. It does not interfere with sleep and the intensity of the pain varies between patients.

Patients with thalamic pain often find that it is exacerbated by cold, fatigue or stress and relieved by relaxation and warmth. This allows them to sleep normally, although they may wake with pain or be woken by it. Treatment modalities that may prove helpful are relaxation and stress management. In some cases ultrasound has also been found to reduce the pain so that treatment of the affected limb can be carried out.

| 12 | **Pain management** |

PHILOSOPHY

The current thinking with regard to pain management is to provide the individual with the tools to manage the pain, not necessarily to cure it. Pain management courses aim to introduce the concept of pain management and to involve the individual in the practical aspects of the course. They also educate course participants in the principles of managing activity through the concepts of pacing and goal setting. They provide information on the processes of pain transmission and regulation so that the individual has a broad overview of the complexities of pain transmission and the concept of the gate control theory of pain. The participants should also have understood the benefits of regular exercise and increased fitness and relaxation technique. Practical sessions include exercise and relaxation. Many programmes include a session on maintenance and setbacks so that the individual is able to cope after the programme is finished. The concepts used are equally applicable when treating pain patients on a one-to-one basis and can be utilized to the benefit of the patient in the treatment process.

Much of the information in this book is based on the author's experience in working in multidisciplinary teams at Gloucestershire Royal Hospital, Gloucester and some work carried out with the pain team at Input, St Thomas' Hospital, London.

PRACTICE

This book has tried to promote a holistic approach to pain management. Many of the complementary therapies can be utilized successfully with both acute and chronic pain. However these methods of pain management should be evaluated and used in terms of the individual's requirements, available facilities and human resources. Ideally a range of therapies is needed in every setting to suit the needs of the individual (Stevenson, 1994). The availability of written information is important as the individual is then able to make an informed choice with regard to treatment.

Currently there is evidence to support the use of many methods of pain management in both acute and chronic pain. These include information-giving, relaxation techniques, distraction, massage, acupuncture, TENS and cognitive behavioural techniques. Other techniques that may be used are biofeedback techniques, aromatherapy, reflexology, shiatsu and hypnosis. However, research into the benefits of these techniques is inconclusive at present.

GUIDELINES

Currently, various professional bodies and multidisciplinary groups are formulating guidelines for practice in both acute and chronic pain. The International Association for the Study of Pain published a document in 1990 on desirable characteristics for pain management treatment facilities in America and Seers *et al.* (1994) are working on guidelines on the establishment of effective pain management facilities and programmes in the UK. Clinical guidelines for the management of acute pain will be published in 1996 by the NHS Executive Nursing Directorate; these guidelines have a multidisciplinary input and cover the management of patients in both hospital and community. Pain management is now a recognized form of treatment and the formulation of guidelines for management and practice will ensure that standards of practice are maintained.

Several of the professions also have special interest groups for pain management. These groups also contribute to standards and guidelines and are keen to ensure a uniformity of practice and to encourage research in this field. The groups form an interprofessional network and communication for professionals working in pain management.

CONCLUSION

Pain management with both acute and chronic patients is a developing area of practice. Pain teams are being established in many parts of the country and there are now several inpatient programmes as well as many outpatient programmes for the treatment of chronic pain. In the field of acute pain it is now recognized that pain control should be suited to the individual patient and that the patient should play an active part in this process. Relaxation and self-medication are being used and TENS machines are becoming more readily available to patients. Information and instruction in self-management of pain is now seen as an important part of patient rehabilitation and in some areas is given as part of the pre-operative process. The development of pain management into a patient-oriented process will ensure that the patient receives information and teaching that will enable them to cope with both acute and chronic pain. This book is only intended as an introduction to the subject of pain management. Those interested in expanding their knowledge further are referred to the reading list below.

FURTHER READING

Carroll, E. and Bowsher, D. (1995) *Pain Management and Nursing Care*, Butterworth-Heinemann, Oxford.

McCaffery, M. and Beebe, A. (1994) *Pain: Clinical Manual for Nursing Practice* (ed. J. Latham), UK edition, C. V. Mosby, London.

Melzack, R. and Wall, P. (1991) *The Challenge of Pain*, Penguin, Harmondsworth.

Wells, P. E., Frampton, V. and Bowsher, D. (1994) *Pain Management by Physiotherapy*, Butterworth-Heinemann, Oxford.

References

Affleck, A., Bianchi, E., Cleckley, M. *et al.* (1984) Stress management as a component of occupational therapy in acute care settings, in *Occupational Therapy and the Patient With Pain*, (ed. F. S. Cromwell), Haworth Press, New York, p. 18.

Alfredsson, L., Spetz, C. L. and Theorell, T. (1985) Type of occupation and near-future hospitalization for myocardial infarction and some other diagnoses. *Int. J. Epidemiol.,* **14**, 378–388.

Arnetz, B. B., Wasserman, J., Petrini, B. *et al.* (1987) Immune function in unemployed women. *Psychosomat. Med.,* **49**, 3–11.

Bandura, A. (1977) Self-efficacy: toward a unifying theory of behavioural change. *Psychol. Rev.,* **84**, 191–215.

Bandura, A. (1982) Self efficacy mechanism in human agency. *Am. Psychol,* **37**, 122–148.

Barker, S. (1978) *The Alexander Technique: The Revolutionary Way to Use Your Body for Total Energy*, Bantam Books, New York.

Beck, A. T. (1987) *Depression: Clinical, Experimental, and Theoretical Aspects*, Harper & Row, New York.

Beck, A. T. and Emery, G. (1985) *Anxiety Disorders and Phobias*, Basic Books, New York.

Beecher, H. K. (1956) Relationship of significance of wound to the pain experienced. *J.A.M.A.,* **161**, 1609–1613..

Beecher, H. K. (1959) *Measurement of Subjective Responses*, Oxford University Press, New York.

Benson, H. (1976) *The Relaxation Response*, William Morrow, New York.

Bergner, M., Bobbitt, R. A., Kressel, S. *et al.* (1976) The sickness impact profile: conceptual formulation and methodology for the development of a health status measure. *Int. J. Health Sci.,* **6**, 393–415.

Bond, M. R. and Pearson, I. B. (1969) Psychological aspects of pain in women with advanced carcinoma of the cervix. *J. Psychosomat. Res.,* **13**, 13–19.

Bonica, J. J. (1980) Cancer pain, in *Pain*, (ed. J. J. Bonica), Raven Press, New York, pp. 335–362.

Bonica, J. J. (ed.) (1990) *The Management of Pain*, 2nd edn, Lea & Febiger, Malvern, PA.

Bonnel, A. M. and Boureau, F. (1985) Labor pain assessment: validity of a behavioural index. *Pain*, **22**, 81–90.

Boring, E. G. (1942) *Sensation and Perception in the History of Experimental Psychology*, Appleton-Century-Crofts, New York.

Bowsher, D. (1986) Pain mechanisms in man. *Medical Times*, **113**, 83–96.

Brown, G. W. and Harris, T. (1978) *Social Origins of Depression: A Study of Psychiatric Disorder in Women*, Tavistock, London.

Cailliet, R. (1991) *Shoulder Pain*, F. A. Davis, Philadelphia, PA.

Cailliet, R. (1992) *Knee Pain and Disability*, F. A. Davis, Philadelphia, PA.

Calvert, R. (1992) A new image for the old adage. *Massage*, **37**, 4.

Cannon, W. B., (1935) Stress and strains of homeostasis. *Am. J. Med. Sci.*, **189**, 1–14.

Carlen, P. L., Wall, P. D., Nadvorna, H. and Steinbach, T. (1978) Phantom limbs and related phenomena in recent traumatic amputations. *Neurology*, **28**, 211–217.

Carroll, D. (1992) *Health Psychology: Stress, Behaviour and Disease*, Falmer Press, London.

Carroll, D. and Bowsher, D. (1995) *Pain Management and Nursing Care*, Butterworth-Heinemann, Oxford.

Carroll, D. and Cross, G. (1990) The academics who double as electricians. *The Independent*, **11 Oct**, p. 23.

Choiniere, M., Melzack, R., Girard, N. *et al.* (1990) Comparisons between patients' and nurses' assessments of pain and medication efficacy in severe burn injuries. *Pain*, **40**, 143–152.

Churcher, M. D. and Ingall, J. R. F. (1987) Sympathetic dependent pain. *Pain Clin.*, **1**, 217–228.

Clarke, A., Allard, L. and Baybrooks, B. A. (1987) *Rehabilitation in Rheumatology. The Team Approach*, Martin Dunitz, London, p. 90.

Collen, M. F., Cutler, J. L., Siegelaub, A. B. and Cella, R. L. (1969) Reliability of the self-administered questionnaire. *Arch. Intern. Med.*, **123**, 664.

Comings, D. E. and Amromin, G. D. (1974) Autosomal dominant insensitivity to pain with hyperplastic myelinopathy and autosomal dominant indifference to pain. *Neurology*, **24**, 838–848.

Copp, L. G. (ed.) (1985) *Perspectives on Pain*, Churchill Livingstone, New York.

Corey, D. T., Etlin, D. and Miller, P. C. (1987) A home-based pain management and rehabilitation programme: an evaluation. *Pain*, **29**, 219–229.

Creek, J. (1990) *Occupational Therapy and Mental Health: Principles, Skills and Practice*, Churchill Livingstone, Edinburgh.

Cyriax, J. H. and Cyriax, P. J. (1984) *The Illustrated Manual of Orthopaedic Medicine*, prepared for Geigy Pharmaceuticals, London.

Dallenbach, K. M. (1939) Pain: history and present status. *Am. J. Psychol.*, **52**, 331–347.

Descartes, R. (1664) *L'Homme*, trans. M. Foster (1901) *Lectures on the History of Physiology during the 16th, 17th and 18th centuries*, Cambridge University Press, Cambridge.

Estlander, A. M. and Harkpaa, K. (1989) Relationships between coping strategies, disability and pain levels in patients with chronic low back pain. *Scand. J. Behav. Ther.*, **18**, 59–69.

Fairbank, C. T., Couper, J., Davies, J. and O'Brien, J. P. (1980) The Oswestry Low Back Pain Disability Questionnaire. *Physiotherapy*, **66**(8).

Fisher, K. (1993) Emotion and perceived control as predictors of disability in chronic pain patients. *J. Pain Soc.*, **11**(1).

Fontana, A. F., Kerns, R. D., Rosenberg, R. L. and Colonese, K. L. (1989) Support, stress and recovery from coronary heart disease: a longitudinal causal model. *Health Psychol.*, **8**, 175–193.

Fordyce, W. E. (1976) *Behavioural Methods for Chronic Pain and Illness*, C. V. Mosby, St Louis, MO.

Fordyce, W. E. (1982) A behavioural perspective on chronic pain, in *Behavioural Medicine* (special issue), *Br. J. Clin. Psych.*, **21**, 75.

Fordyce, W. E. (1984) Behavioural science and chronic pain. *Postgrad. Med. J.*, **60**, 865–868.

Fordyce, W. E., Caldwell, L. and Hongadarin, T. (1979) Effects of performance feedback on exercise tolerance in chronic pain. Unpublished manuscript, University of Washington, Seattle, WA.

Fridh, G., Kopare, T., Gaston-Johansson, F. and Norvell, K. T. (1988) Factors associated with more intense labor pain. *Res. Nurs. Health*, **11**, 117–124.

Friedman, M., Thoresen, C. E., Gill, J. J. *et al.* (1986) Alteration of Type A behaviour and its effects on cardiac recurrences in postmyocardial infarction patients: summary of the Recurrent Coronary Prevention Project. *Am. Heart J.*, **112**, 653–665.

Fulder, S. and Munro, R. (1982) *The Status of Complementary Medicine in the UK*, Threshold Foundation, London.

Glass, D. C. and Singer, J. E. (1972) *Urban Stress*, Academic Press, New York.

Grant, B. (1993) *A–Z of Natural Healthcare*, Optima. London.

Guyton, A. C. (1981) *Basic Human Neurophysiology*, W. B. Saunders, Philadelphia, PA.

Hall, K. R. L. and Stride, E. (1954) The varying response to pain in psychiatric disorders: a study in abnormal psychology. *Br. J. Med. Psychol.*, **27**, 48–60.

Halliday, T., Robinson, D., Stirling, V. *et al.* (1992) Book 3, The Senses and Communication, in *Biology: Brain and Behaviour*, Open University, Milton Keynes.

Hardy, P. A. J. and Hill, P. (1990) A multidisciplinary approach to pain management. *Br. J. Hosp. Med.*, **43**, 45–47.

Harvey, P. (1988) *Health Psychology*, Longman, Harlow.

Hayne, C. R. (1987) *Total Back Care*, J. M. Dent & Sons, London.

Hazard, R. G., Fenwick, J. W., Kalisch, S. M. *et al.* (1989) Functional restoration with behavioural support. *Spine*, **14**(2), 157–161.

Head, H. (1920) *Studies in Neurology*, Kegan Paul, London.

Hewitt, J. (1985) *Teach Yourself Relaxation*, Hodder & Stoughton, London.

Hodges, C. and Bender, L. (1994) Phantom pain: a critical review of the proposed mechanisms. *Br. J. Occ. Ther.*, **57**(6).

Hokanson, J. E., DeGood, D. E., Forest, M. S. and Brittain, T. M. (1971) Availability of avoidance behaviours in modulating vascular-stress responses. *J. Personality Soc. Psychol.*, **19**, 60–68.

Holmes, J. A. and Stephenson, C. A. Z. (1990) Differential effects of avoidant and attentional coping strategies on adaptation to chronic and recent-onset pain. *Health Psychol.*, **9**, 577–584.

Hosobuchi, Y., Adams, J. E. and Linchitz, R. (1977) Pain relief by electrical stimulation of the central grey matter in humans and its reversal by naloxone. *Science*, **177**, 183–186.

Houde, R. W. (1982) Methods for measuring clinical pain in humans. *Acta. Anaesth. Scand. Suppl.*, **74**, 25–29.

House, J. S., McMichael, A. J., Wells, J. A. *et al.* (1979) Occupational stress and health among factory workers. *J. Health Soc. Behav.*, **20**, 139–160.

International Association for the Study of Pain (1990) *Desirable Characteristics for Pain Treatment Facilities*, I. A. S. P., Seattle, WA.

Jackson, T. (1991) An evaluation of the Mitchell method of simple physiological relaxation for women with rheumatoid arthritis. *Br. J. Occ. Ther.*, **54**(3).

Jacobson, E. (1929) *Progressive Relaxation*, University of Chicago Press, Chicago, IL.

Jacobson, E. (1962) *You Must Relax*, McGraw-Hill, New York.

Jakubowski-Spector, P. (1973) Facilitating the growth of women through assertive training. *Counselling Psychologist*, **4**, 75–86.

Jensen, M. P., Karoly, P. and Braver, S. (1986) The measurement of clinical pain intensity: a comparison of six methods. *Pain*, **27**, 117–126.

Jensen, T. S., Krebs, B., Nielson, J. and Rasmussen, P. (1983) Phantom limb, phantom pain and stump pain in amputees during the first six months following limb amputation. *Pain*, **17**, 243–256.

Jensen, T. S., Krebs, B., Nielson, J. and Rasmussen, P. (1985) Immediate and long term phantom limb pain in amputees: incidence, clinical characteristics and relationship to pre-amputation limb pain. *Pain*, **21**, 267–278.

Jette, A. M. (1985) State of the art in functional status assessment, in *Measurement in Physical Therapy*, (ed. J. Rothstein), Churchill Livingstone, New York, p. 140.

Kavanagh, J. (1995) Management of chronic pain using the cognitive-behavioural approach. *Br. J. Ther. Rehab.*, **2**(8).

Keable, D. (1985) Relaxation training techniques: a review. Part two: how effective is relaxation training? *Br. J. Occ. Ther.*, **48**(7), 201–204.

Keable, D. (1989) *The Management of Anxiety*, Churchill Livingstone, Edinburgh.

Keefe, F. J. and Block, A. R. (1982) Development of an observation method for assessing pain behaviour in chronic low back pain patients. *Behav. Ther.*, **13**, 363–375.

Keefe, F. J. and Williams, D. A. (1989) New directions in pain assessment and treatment. *Clin. Psychol. Rev.*, **9**, 549–568.

Keele, K. D. (1957) *Anatomies of Pain*, Oxford University Press, Oxford.

Larbig, W. (1982) *Schmerz: Grundlagen; Forsching; Therapie*, W. Kohlhammer, Stuttgart.

Lavies, N., Hart, L., Rounsefell, B. and Runciman, W. (1992) Identification of patient, medical and nursing staff attitudes to post-operative opioid analgesia: stage 1 of a longitudinal study of post operative analgesia. *Pain*, **48**, 313–319.

Lazarus, R. S. and Cohen, J. B. (1977) Environmental stress, in *Human Behaviour and the Environment: Current Theory and Research* (eds I. Attman and J. F. Wohlwill), Plenum Press, New York.

Lazarus, R. S. and Folkman, S. (1984) *Stress, Appraisal and Coping*, Springer, New York.

Lazarus, R. S., Opton, E. M. Jr, Nomikos, M. S. and Rankin, N. O. (1965) The principle of short-circuiting threat: further evidence. *J. Personality*, **33**, 622–635.

Levenson, C. (1971) Rehabilitation of the stroke hemiplegia patient, in *Handbook of Physical Medicine and Rehabilitation* (eds F. H. Krusen, F. J. Kottke and P. M. Ellwood), W. B. Saunders, Philadelphia, PA.

Lipton, S. (1979) The treatment of chronic pain, in *The Control of Chronic Pain*, (ed. S. Lipton), Edward Arnold, London, ch. 10.

Livingston, W. K. (1943) *Pain Mechanisms*, Macmillan, New York.

Loeser, J. D. (1980) Low back pain, in *Pain* (ed. J. J. Bonica), Raven Press, New York, p. 367–377.

McCaffery, M. and Beebe, A. (1989) *Pain: Clinical Manual for Nursing Practice*, C. V. Mosby, Toronto.

McCaul, K. D. and Malott, J. (1984) Distraction and coping with pain. *Psychol. Bull.*, **95**, 516–553.

Mackarness, R. (1976) *Not All in the Mind*, Pan, London.

McQuay, H. J. (1990) Assessment of pain, and effectiveness of treatment, in *Measuring the Outcomes of Medical Care*, (eds A. Hopkins and D Costain).

Marino, J., Gwynn M. I. and Spanos, N. I. (1989) Cognitive mediators in the reduction of pain: the role of expectancy, strategy use, and self-presentation. *J. Abnorm. Psych.*, **98**(3), 256–262.

Marshall, H. R. (1894) *Pain, Pleasure and Aesthetics*, Macmillan, London.

Martin, P. R., Nathan, P. R., Milech, D. and Van Keppel, M. (1989) Cognitive therapy vs. self management training in treatment of chronic headaches. *Br. J. Clin. Psych.*, **28**, 347–361.

Mather, L. and Mackie, J. (1983) The incidence of postoperative pain in children. *Pain*, **15**, 271–282.

Max, M. P., Portonoy, R. K. and Laska, E. M. (eds) (1991) Advances in pain research and therapy, in *The Design of Analgesic Clinical Trials*, Raven Press, New York.

Mayer, D. J., Wolfe, T. L., Akil, H. *et al.* (1971) Analgesia from electrical stimulation in the brainstem of the rat. *Science*, **174**, 1351–1354.

Mayer, T. G., Gatchel, R. J., Mayer, H. *et al.* (1987) A prospective two year study of functional restoration in industrial low back injury utilizing objective assessment. *J.A.M.A.*, **258**, 1763–1767.

Meichenbaum, D. (1977) *Cognitive Behavioural Modification*, Plenum Press, New York.

Melzack, R. (1987) The short form McGill Pain Questionnaire. *Pain*, **30**, 191–197.

Melzack, R. and Casey, K. L. (1968) Sensory, motivational and central control determinants of pain: a new conceptual model, in *The Skin Senses*, (ed. D. Kenshalo), Charles C. Thomas, Springfield, IL, p. 423–443.

Melzack, R. and Wall, P. D. (1965) Pain mechanisms: a new theory. *Science*, **150**, 971–979.

Melzack, R. and Wall, P. D. (1991) *The Challenge of Pain*, Penguin, Harmondsworth.

Melzack, R., Abbott, F. V., Zackon, W. *et al.* (1987) Pain on a surgical ward: a survey of the duration and intensity of pain and the effectiveness of medication. *Pain*, **29**, 67–72.

Melzack, R., Guite, S. and Gonshor, A. (1980) Relief of dental pain by ice massage of the hand. *Can. Med. Assoc. J.*, **122**, 189–191.

Melzack, R., Wall, P. D. and Ty, T. C. (1982) Acute pain in an emergency clinic: latency of onset and descriptor patterns. *Pain*, **14**, 33–43.

Mitchell, S. W. (1872) *Injuries of Nerves and Their Consequences*, J. B. Lippincott, Philadelphia, PA.

Mitchell, S. W., Morehouse, C. R. and Keen, W. W. (1864) *Gunshot Wounds and Other Injuries of the Nerve*, J. B. Lippincott, Philadelphia, PA.

Mowrer, O. H. and Vick, P. (1948) An experimental analogue of fear from a sense of helplessness. *J. Abnorm. Soc. Psychol.*, **43**, 193–200.

Muller, J. (1842) *Elements of Physiology*, Taylor, London.

Murphy, T. M. (1987) Treatment of intractable pain. *Ann. Acad. Med. Singapore*, **16**(2), 256–260.

Nashold, B. S., Higgins, A. C. and Blumenkopf, B. (1985) Dorsal root entry zone lesions for pain relief, in *Neurosurgery*, vol. 3, (eds R. S. Wilkins and S. S. Rengachary), McGraw-Hill, New York, p. 2433–2437.

Nathan, P. W. and Wall, P. D. (1974) Treatment of post-herpetic neuralgia by prolonged electrical stimulation. *Br. Med. J.*, 3, 645–647.

Niven, C. (1986) Factors affecting labour pain. Unpublished PhD thesis, University of Stirling, Stirling.

Niven, C. and Gijsbers, K. (1984) A study of labor pain using the McGill pain questionnaire. *Soc. Sci. Med.*, **19**, 1347–1351.

Noback, C. R. and Demarest, R. (1977) *The Nervous System, Introduction and Review*, 2nd edn, McGraw Hill, New York.

Noordenbos, W. (1959) *Pain*, Elsevier, Amsterdam.

O'Hara, P. M. (1990) The pain for which there is no cure. *Ther. Weekly*, **11 Oct.**

Olesen, J. (1986) The pathophysiology of migraine, in *Handbook of Clinical Neurology*, vol. 48, rev. series (ed. F. C. Rose), Elsevier, Amsterdam, p. 59–83.

Orth-Gomer, K. M. and Unden, A. L. (1990) Type A behaviour, social support and coronary risk: interaction and significance for mortality in cardiac patients. *Psychosomat. Med.*, **52**, 59–72.

Painter, J. R., Seres, J. L. and Newman, R. I. (1980) Assessing benefits of the pain center: why some patients regress. *Pain*, **8**, 101–113.

Partridge, C. J. and Johnston, M. (1989) Perceived control and recovery from stroke. *Br. J. Clin. Psychol.*, **28**, 53–60.

Patt, R. B. and Balter, K. (1991) Post traumatic reflex sympathetic dystrophy: mechanisms and medical management. *J. Occ. Rehab.*, **1**(1).

Pavlov, I. P. (1927) *Conditioned Reflexes*, Humphrey Milford, Oxford.

Pavlov, I. P. (1928) *Lectures on Conditioned Reflexes*, International Publishers, New York.

Pearce, C. (1995) Care of the dying, in *Pain Management and Nursing Care*, (eds D. Carroll and D. Bowsher), Butterworth-Heinemann, Oxford.

Pearson, R. M. (1990) *Muscle Overuse Syndrome*, The Musicians' and Keyboard Clinic, London.

Pedretti, L. W. (1985) *Occupational Therapy: Practice Skills for Physical Dysfunction*, C. V. Mosby, St Louis, MO.

Pedretti, L. W. and Zoltan, B. (1990) *Occupational Therapy: Practice Skills for Physical Dysfunction*, 3rd edn, C. V. Mosby, St Louis, MO.

Pert, C. B. and Snyder, S. H. (1973) Opiate receptor: demonstration in nervous tissue. *Science*, **179**, 1011–1014.

Phillips, K. (1988) Strategies against AIDS. *Psychologist*, **Feb.**, p. 46–47.

Pikoff, H. (1984) Is the muscular model of headache still viable? A review of conflicting data. *Headache*, **24**, 186–198.

Pinsky, J. J. (1983) Psychodynamic understanding and treatment of the chronic intractable benign pain syndrome – treatment outcome. *Semin. Neurol.*, **3**, 346–354.

Polgar, S. and Thomas, S. A. (1991) *Introduction to Research in the Health Sciences*, Churchill Livingstone, Edinburgh.

Rahe, R. H. (1975) Life changes and near-future illness reports, in *Emotions: Their Parameters and Measurements*, (ed. L. Levi), Raven Press, New York.

Ralphs, J. (1995) The cognitive behavioural treatment of chronic pain, in *Pain Management and Nursing Care*, (eds D. Carroll and D. Bowsher) Butterworth-Heinemann, Oxford.

Read, A. E. and Cox, D. N. (1985) Psychosocial predictors of labor pain. *Pain*, **22**, 309–315.

Reed, K. and Sanderson, S. (1983) *Concepts of Occupational Therapy*, Williams & Wilkins, Baltimore, MD.

Reese, L. (1983) Coping with pain: the role of perceived self-efficacy (doctoral dissertation, Stanford University). *Dissertation Abstracts International*, **44**, 1641B.

Richardson, I. H., Richardson, P. H., Williams, A. C. de C. *et al.* (1994) The effects of a cognitive-behavioural pain management programme on the quality of work and employment status of severely impaired chronic pain patients. *Disabil. Rehab.*, **16**(1), 26–34.

Rim, D. C. and Masters, J. C. (1974) Behaviour Therapy: Techniques and Empirical Findings, Academic Press, New York.

Rosenhan, D. L. (1973) On being sane in insane places. *Science*, **179**, 250–268.

Roth, I. (ed.) (1990) *Introduction to Psychology*, vol. 2, Open University, Lawrence Erlbaum Associates.

Roth, I. and Frisby, J. P. (1989) *Perception and Representation: A Cognitive Approach*, Open Guides to Psychology, Open University Press, Milton Keynes.

Royal College of Surgeons of England and the College of Anaesthetists (1990) *Report of the Working Party on Pain After Surgery*, RCS, London.

Royle, J. A. and Walsh, M. (1992) *Watson's Medico-Surgical Nursing and Related Physiology*, 4th edn, Baillière Tindall, London.

Saunders, C. (1989) *The Management of Terminal Malignant Disease*, 2nd edn., Edward Arnold, London.

Schmidt, A. J. M. (1985a) Cognitive factors in the performance level of chronic low back pain patients. *J. Psychosomat. Res.*, **29**, 183–189.

Schmidt, A. J. M. (1985b) Performance level of chronic low back pain patients in different treadmill conditions. *J. Psychosomat. Res.*, **29**, 639–645.

Schott, G. D. (1986) Mechanisms of causalgia and related clinical conditions. *Brain*, **109**, 717–738.

Schultz, J. H. and Luthe, W. (1969) *Autogenic Therapy*, vols 1–5, Grune & Stratton, New York.

Schwartz, D. P., DeGood, D. E. and Shutty, M. S. (1985) Direct assessment of beliefs and attitudes of chronic pain patients. *Arch. Phys. Med. Rehab.*, **66**, 806–809.

Seers, K., Williams, A. C. de C., Richardson, P. *et al.* (1994) Draft guidelines on the establishment of effective pain management facilities and programmes.

Selye, H. (1956) *The Stress of Life*, McGraw-Hill, New York.

Sensky, T. (1990) Patients' reactions to illness. *Br. Med. J.*, **300**, 622–623.

Sherman, R. A. (1994) What do we really know about phantom limb pain? *Pain Reviews*, **1**(4).

Shutty, M. S., DeGood, D. E. and Hoekstra, D. M. (1987) Assessment of chronic pain patients beliefs about rehabilitative strategies: relationship to coping styles and treatment outcome (abstract). *Pain Suppl.*, **4**, S326.

Snyder, S. H. (1977) Opiate receptors and internal opiates. *Sci. Am.*, **236**, 44–56.

Sofaer, B. (1992) *Pain: A Handbook for Nurses*, Chapman & Hall, London.

Staub, E., Tursky, B. and Schwartz, G. E. (1971) Self-control and predictability: the effects on reactions to aversive stimulation. *J. Personality Soc. Psychol.*, **18**, 157–162.

Sternbach, R. A. (1982) The psychologist's role in the diagnosis and treatment of pain patients, in *Psychological Approaches to the Management of Pain*, (eds J. Barber and C. Adrian), Brunner Mazal, ch. 1.

Sternbach, R. A. and Timmermans, G. (1975) Personality changes associated with reduction of pain. *Pain*, **1**, 177–181.

Sternbach, R. A. and Tursky, B. (1965) Ethnic differences among housewives in psychophysical and skin potential responses to electric shock. *Psychophysiology*, **1**, 241–246.

Stevenson, C. J. (1994) *Non-pharmacological Aspects of Acute Pain Management*, Consensus Conference to develop guidelines for acute pain management. NHS Nursing Directorate, London.

Strong, J. (1991) Relaxation training and chronic pain. *Br. J. Occ. Ther.*, **54**(6), 216–218.

Suls, J. and Fletcher, B. (1985) The relative efficacy of avoidant and nonavoidant coping strategies: a met-analysis. *Health Psychol.*, **4**, 249–288.

Sutherland, J. E., Wesley, R. M., Cole, P. M. *et al.* (1988) Differences and similarities between patient and physician perceptions of pain. *Fam. Med.*, **20**, 343–346.

Svensson, J. and Theorell, T. (1983) Life events and elevated blood pressure in young men. *J. Psychosomat. Res.*, **27**, 445–456.

Swanson, D. W., Swenson, W. M., Maruta, T. and McPhee, M. C. (1976) Program for managing chronic pain. *Proc. Staff Meetings Mayo Clinic*, **51**, 401–408.

Tanner, J. (1987) *Beating Back Pain: A Practical Self-Help Guide to Prevention and Treatment*, Dorling Kindersley, London.

Taylor, C. B., Zlutnick, S. I., Corley, M. J. and Flora, J. (1980) The effects of detoxification, relaxation and brief supportive therapy on chronic pain. *Pain*, **8**, 303–318.

Taylor, H. and Curran, N. M. (1985) *The Nuprin Pain Report*, Louis Harris, New York.

Theorell, T., Knox, S., Svensson, J. and Waller, D. (1985) Blood pressure variations during a working day at age 28: effects of different types of work and blood pressure levels at age 18. *J. Hum. Stress*, **11**, 36–41.

Twycross, R. G. and Lack, S. A. (1990) *Therapeutics in Terminal Care*, Churchill Livingstone, Edinburgh.

Urban, B. J. and Nashold, B. S. (1978) Percutaneous epidural stimulation of the spinal cord for relief of pain. *J. Neurosurg.*, **48**, 323–328.

Vlaeyen, J. W. S., Snijders, A. M. J., Schuerman, J. A. *et al.* (1989) Chronic pain and the three systems model of emotions, a critical examination. *Tijdschr.-Psychiatr.*, **31**(2), 100–113.

Vlaeyen, J. W. S., Snijders, A. M., Scheurman, J. A. *et al.* (1990) What do chronic pain patients think of their pain? Towards a pain cognition questionnaire. *Br. J. Clin. Psychol.*, **29**(4), 383–394.

Waddell, G., Bircher, M., Finlayson, D. and Main, C. J. (1984) Symptoms and signs: physical disease or illness behaviour? *Br. Med. J.*, **289**, 739–741.

Wall, P. D. (1960) Cord cells responding to touch, damage and temperature of skin. *J. Neurophysiol.*, **23**, 197–210.

Wall, P. D. (1981) On the origin of pain associated with amputation, in *Phantom and Stump Pain*, (eds J. Siegfried and M. Zimmermann), Springer-Verlag, Berlin, p. 2–14.

Watts, C. (1985) Chemonucleolysis, in *Neurosurgery*, vol. 3, (eds R. H. Wilkins and S. S. Rengachary), McGraw-Hill, New York, p. 2260–2264.

Weddell, G. (1955) Somesthesis and the chemical senses. *Annu. Rev. Psychol.*, **6**, 119–136.

Williams, D. and Thorn, B. (1989) An empirical assessment of pain beliefs. *Pain*, **36**, 351–358.

Wolpe, J. and Lange, P. J. (1964) A fear schedule for use in behaviour therapy. *Behav. Res. Ther.*, **2**, 27–30.

Working Party (1993) Anaesthetists and non-acute pain management. The Association of Anaesthetists of Great Britain and Ireland, the Royal College of Anaesthetists and the Pain Society, London.

Wynn Parry, C. B. (1980) Pain in avulsion lesions of the brachial plexus. *Pain*, **9**, 41–53.

Zalon, M. L. (1993) Nurse's assessment of post-operative patient's pain. *Pain*, **54**, 329–334.

Zborowski, M. (1969) *People in Pain*, Jossey-Bass, San Francisco, CA.

Index